Healthcare EQ

Healthcare EQ

A Clinician's Guide

Robert Driver, MD
& Dr. Izzy Justice

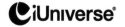

HEALTHCARE EQ
A Clinician's Guide

iUniverse books may be ordered through booksellers or by contacting:

iUniverse
1663 Liberty Drive
Bloomington, IN 47403
www.iuniverse.com
1-800-Authors (1-800-288-4677)

ISBN: 978-1-5320-4170-9 (sc)
ISBN: 978-1-5320-4263-8 (hc)
ISBN: 978-1-5320-4171-6 (e)

Library of Congress Control Number: 2018900748

Print information available on the last page.

iUniverse rev. date: 01/26/2018

Dedication

To Zoe and Griffin, my motivation to be my best. And to my patients who have allowed me into their lives. *-Dr. Driver*

To Stephanie, Lexi, Hunter, and my eternal mentor, Gary Mason. *-Dr. Justice*

Acknowledgments

This book would not be possible without the invaluable input from several people, and we are grateful to everyone involved. Special thanks go to Judah Lindenburg, MD, for providing such an insightful foreword. Many thanks to Bimal Shah, MD, for all the assistance, and to the following people for all their written endorsements: David Voran, MD; Jeffrey Rose, MD; Michael Ash, MD, FACP; Paula Evans, MSN, RN, CEN; Doreen McCormick, MSPT, INHC; Michael Frye, MD, FACEP; Sarah Scibetta, RN; Dina Khentigan, MSN, RN, C-EFM, CPFI. Finally, we would also like to express much thanks to our editor, Anjum Khan.

Contents

Foreword

Emotional Intelligence (EQ) is perplexing to many, not so much because it's so hard to understand, but rather because of how easily it is misunderstood. As Chief of Staff at my hospital, I have encountered this bit of misapprehension in my colleagues, my staff, and myself; and it's a serious barrier to personal growth.

As I grew into the role, I kept track of some important guidelines which emerged as critical tools for discharging my responsibilities and negotiating change and conflict. I've written some codes of management for myself. Amongst those (the list is now over forty) rules are:

- Don't judge until you know the facts
- Don't become part of the drama
- Ask yourself, "What is the outcome I want?"
- Presume that you have something to learn
- Don't burn bridges
- Pick your battles AND your moments

Many would categorize these behaviors as merely being nice and caring, or common sense, or an effortless expression of empathy, but they would be wrong. What they all share is their reliance on the active application of emotional intelligence. EQ manifests itself in both the workplace and life as it is the ability to listen, manage conflict, and collaborate to solve problems. It infuses a person with confidence, self-control, and the ability to inspire and influence others.

One of the most frustrating myths encountered about EQ is the belief that a person either has it or does not. This binary assertion is tantamount to saying that it's a skill one cannot learn, that only those who received the gift at birth are capable of it. Rather, it is like almost every other skill in life. It can be developed. It may come as a shock to most people that despite being a physician, I don't play golf. I've never touched a golf club let alone played a round. As such, I can guarantee my first go at it would be a fair bit worse than Michael Jordan playing professional baseball; but, I also expect that if I took lessons and devotedly practiced, I could eventually become respectable. I might not demonstrate Tiger Woods' ability, but I would be much better than I am now. EQ training is much the same, and this book can help you harness whatever innate measure of EQ you possess and stimulate its growth, especially as a clinician in healthcare.

What makes *this* book about EQ so valuable is that it's not just a recitation of parables or a list of self-help techniques. It engages the reader to be a proactive participant and driver of the transformation that will come while developing one's emotional intelligence. In a real sense, it inspires the reader to become a determined participant rather than a passive receptacle.

Everything you need to awaken your EQ spirit lies within. Beginning with a focus on self-awareness, the very foundation of emotional intelligence, the authors train the reader to recruit often untapped senses to the task. They demonstrate how critical EQ is to everyday decision making – at every level – and describe the neuroscience of the limbic system to elucidate how easy it is for the amygdala to hijack a cognitive process and cause undesired outcomes. In turn, they demonstrate how to counter the emotional currents, first by recognizing them and then by exerting conscious control; and they provide a rigorous framework for both short and long-term success.

Becoming emotionally intelligent is a choice, not a birthright. From the autist to the empath, virtually everyone has a measure of it. Dr. Driver gives credence to this claim with a poignantly personal story of his own enlightenment in Chapter 6. The same awakening awaits us all, if we only agree to give up the passive acceptance of emotional tone deafness and decide to embrace the potential which lies within us all. The stakes are now higher than ever for physicians in particular.

Practicing medicine has long been a high-stress endeavor. As the authors point out, burnout is looming ominously over the future of healthcare. It threatens a physician shortage, as affected doctors retire early or switch into non-clinical roles at a time when demand for medical care is higher than ever. Manufacturing new physicians is analogous to producing bourbon. It takes years to get the finished product, meaning that we can't just decide to make more today and have them practice next week. We also now realize that burnout leads to disengagement, which worsens patient outcomes. In moral terms then, you not only *should* read this book, you *need* to read this book.

Judah R. Lindenberg, MD
Chief of Staff
Cleveland Clinic – Marymount Hospital

Introduction

Having worked in the healthcare industry for a combined over 50 years, we have worked with healthcare providers and administrators in a myriad of disciplines. As a physician, or consultant, working with technology, strategy, operations, supply chain or clinical projects, we have witnessed the emotional drain of Clinicians and the organizational infrastructure. Provider institutions are replete with kind, compassionate, and skilled folks who genuinely care about their patients and, in the moment, will do anything for the patient. It is extremely rewarding to leave a shift feeling you have genuinely impacted the life of another human being.

Yet Clinicians struggle on a daily basis with the emotional toll that comes with each patient and his/her family. There is also the stressful dynamic of any workplace of working with peers who have different skills and priorities, as each person comes with a set of unique emotional skills to cope with the grind. We have found a disturbing, but fixable, deficiency in the emotional literacy of people in general, whereby most folks do not even have a language to process emotions.

The concept of professional burnout has been around since 1974, when it was first described and studied by Herbert Freudenberger.

- In 2007, the Department of Health & Human Services (HHS) described professional burnout as a risk that may cause high quality professionals to leave the medical field altogether.
- A national study from 2011, published in the Archives of Internal Medicine, found that 38% of physicians experienced burnout compared to 28% of workers in other industries.

- In 2013, Medscape reported physician burnout rate to be 40% when it was included in their annual survey. This problem has continued to escalate. In the 2017 Medscape survey, 51% of physicians reported experiencing frequent or constant feelings of burnout, revealing a 25% increase in just 4 years.
- According to US news and world reports, physicians have a 10%-20% higher divorce rate than the general population.
- Physicians are also 15 times more likely to experience burnout than professionals in any other line of work.
- Nearly 50% of physicians believe overwork, stress, and fatigue among their colleagues significantly contributes to medical errors, according to a 2014 study in the NEJM.

To set further context for the size and complexity of this industry, consider the recent data below that should alert all of us to the urgency of incorporating EQ into the Clinician skillset.

From source: National Center for Health Statistics.

- Life expectancy at birth is 78.8 for total US population.
- Aging population: "By 2030, it is projected that one in five Americans will be 65 or older."
- Diseases:
  - o 74% of the 2.7 million deaths in 2015 were due to 10 leading causes: heart disease, cancer, chronic lower respiratory diseases, unintentional injuries, stroke, Alzheimer's disease, diabetes, influenza and pneumonia, kidney disease, and suicide.
  - o heart disease and cancer are top 2 leading causes of death (45% of all deaths).
  - o "Smoking is the leading cause of preventable disease, disability, and death."
  - o Obesity is a significant risk factor for numerous chronic diseases and conditions including cardiovascular disease,

diabetes, and cancer. Obesity is a major public health challenge for U.S. and many other countries.
o Diabetes was the 7th leading cause of death in 2015. In 2011–2014, approximately 1 in 9 adults in the United States had diabetes.

- Health expenditure:
  o 17.8% of the U.S. Gross Domestic Product (GDP) was spent on national health care.
  o $2.7 trillion was spent on personal health care for an average of $8,468 per person.
  o In 2014, $186 billion was spent on mental health treatment, representing 6.4% of all health spending & $34 billion was spent on substance use disorder treatment, representing 1.2% of all health spending.
  o the Medicare program covered 55.3 million people.
  o 75% of all health care dollars are spent on patients with one or more chronic conditions, many of which can be prevented, including diabetes, obesity, heart disease, lung disease, high blood pressure, and cancer.
  o 62% of all bankruptcy filings in the United States in 2007 were due to illness or medical bills.

From source: http://www.cdc.gov/nchs/nhis.htm.

- Health Expenses & Insurance:
  o In 2016, 9% of Americans were without any health insurance.
  o 4.4% of the population failed to obtain needed medical care due to cost at some time.
  o The United States is the only wealthy, industrialized nation that does not have a universal health care system.
  o 2.5 million young adults gained health insurance as a result of the Affordable Care Act that allows them to remain on their parents' insurance plans until age 26.

- Diseases & General Population Well-Being:
  - 51.7% (just over half) of U.S. adults aged 18 and over met the 2008 federal physical activity guidelines for aerobic activity (based on leisure-time activity).
  - 25.0% of adults aged 18 and over had at least 1 heavy drinking day in the past year.
  - Only 66.4% of population reported excellent or very good health.
  - 3.6% of adults aged 18 and over had experienced serious psychological distress during the past 30 days of the survey.
  - 8.6% of population had asthma.

From source: Kaiser Family Foundation State Health Facts

- Hospitals:
  - As of 2014, a total of 4,926 hospitals were registered in the U.S.
  - More than 58% of all U.S. hospitals are nonprofit.
  - About 20% of all U.S. hospitals are owned by state or local governments.
  - For-profit hospitals represent 21.4% of all U.S. hospitals.
  - U.S. hospitals see an average of $2,212 adjusted expenses per inpatient day.
  - The average length of stay for inpatient care is 4.8 days.
  - About 7% of patients stay overnight at the hospital.

- Physicians:
  - As of April 2015, there were a total of 908,508 professionally active physicians in the U.S.
  - Nearly 48% of physicians are primary care.
  - About 52% of physicians are specialists.

- Insurance:
  - 49% of the U.S. population is insured through employers.
  - 32% are insured under Medicaid and Medicare.
  - Medicaid costs totaled nearly $500 billion in 2014.

It is easy to forget in all the healthcare statistics and debate that providing care is as much an emotional endeavor as it is a physiological one, or a financial one, for both the patient and the Clinician. On either side of these stakeholders are family members filled with anxiety and administrators working to create a set of transactions that facilitate providing data and resources to Clinicians whilst managing the 'customer' process of being a patient. It is even easier to forget that when each Clinician goes home, he or she takes along the emotional toll of the day. Burnout is an all too common symptom with even the most dedicated professionals.

There seems to be a binary choice for Clinicians: Do what you love to do or have a healthy post-work life. The good news is that with a higher level of emotional intelligence, a learnable competency, and a communal support system within the healthcare institution, it does not have to be choice or compromise. Both can be achieved.

Patients and their families are human beings, just as co-workers and supervisors are. Each brings a set of experiences and very different levels of skill functionally in what is required, but not in managing emotions in chaos. So, it is not just one's own emotions as a Clinician that is critical to manage, but of all these people as well. This makes healthcare a very emotionally challenging environment. Some may argue that other industries face the same challenges, like airlines, hotels, or restaurants with constant flow of customers. Sure, there is stress in these environments, but the fundamental – and hopefully obvious – distinction is that healthcare has customers that are sick. They have family waiting in the hallways for constant updates, and expecting reassurances. There are more regulations that Clinicians have to follow before, during, and after care than arguably any industry, with a lawsuit waiting for even the slightest mishap. An unhappy hotel guest can be given a free night or meal and feel satisfied. Airlines can offer a free trip or an upgrade. Clinicians have no such recourse. They have to get it right the first time, often with incomplete patient information and the clock ticking. A mishap's consequence is usually accompanied with grief and trauma for the Clinicians too. *What else could we have done?* is all too frequent a response to mishaps.

What makes healthcare the ultimate emotional test is all of this coupled with inadequate EQ skills.

The purpose of this book is to address this. A Clinician needs to be at his/her best from the very first patient of the shift till the last one. He/she does not have the luxury of getting drained half way through the day as each patient requires an equally complete and mindful presence of the Clinician, so that all the medical skills can be effectively used to provide the best care with the necessary compassion.

Patients, like most human beings, want to know that a Clinician genuinely cares first, before they care about what the Clinician wants or prescribes. This is an emotional connection they are looking for. Nothing feels as cold and harsh to a patient than feeling like they are just another patient going through a system, like a car in a garage assembly line. Some Clinicians wrestle with a perceived binary choice – *if I show compassion and bond with my patient, will I lose my ability to be objective?* This argument is admission of low EQ as the two can effectively co-exist. Some Clinicians fear showing emotions with all patients is impossible and not necessary. Again, this is a false equivalence founded in low EQ. The contrary is, in fact, true. It is possible that each patient has the potential to replete emotional energy, instead of depleting it, so that EQ is sustained throughout the shift and later at home. We acknowledge this is not how most Clinicians operate and all the more reason to read on.

The central premise of this book is that healthcare is as much an emotional endurance test as it is a medical competency test.

If you do not believe this, then this book will be of little value to you. If you do, then the next logical questions should be: *What do I do to prepare for the emotional endurance test? What can I do to prepare for my work day? What can I do for my peers and my institution? What can I do for my patients?*

In this book, we introduce you to a sequence of mental and emotional preparation, before, during, and after a shift/situation. You will be introduced to a new mental and emotional language similar to the medical language used for your area of expertise. In the latter, Clinicians know what a chart is, various medications, pathologies, a differential diagnosis, diagnostic tests, and technical procedures. These are all words that form a language that allow them to understand the medical dimensions of their job.

In addition to a new language, you will build your own personal game plan. No two human beings are the same mentally and emotionally, so the plan for each person will be different and has to accommodate the emotional fluctuations of both personal and work life, where highs and lows can impact so much of decision-making.

During each shift, the sheer volume of monologues that occur is quite unprecedented. Each monologue, that self-talk, after almost every interaction, is a natural human response to the stimuli of the ever-changing environment, constant flow of patients, and changing staff. We are talking about a totally unique environment that will challenge your emotions to the core.

These emotions, both good and not so good, will dictate the tone and content of the monologues and critical subsequent decision-making. In Chapter 1, we share several stories that almost all Clinicians will be able to relate to where emotions got in the way of the best care.

Yet despite powerful personal stories of underperformance and many more well-documented ones in case studies, the average Clinician still spends almost zero time training his or her emotions and thoughts. We researched dozens of healthcare training programs and videos and found very few that had budgeted time for this kind of training.

One of the first questions that we ask Clinicians is: "What is the most stressful patient situation?" The most common answers we get are "difficult or rude patients", "angry families", and "unrealistic expectations", when faced with mounting external pressures. **It is our absolute contention that the most challenging patient experience for a Clinician is the one right after a bad one**. Why? As we explain in Chapter 2, right after a bad experience, the emotional temperature is so high that cognitive decision-making is neurologically compromised, leading to a very low probability that you can either make the right next decision or cognitively process the right set of protocols with any semblance of compassion.

This is the reason to write this book. We believe that most Clinicians are grossly under training in an area that has the potential to be a game-changer in performance and career longevity. The inexplicable reason, we believe, that very good, competent, intelligent, and hard-working Clinicians are under trained in this area is simply that they do not know how to do it. If it is done, it is done anecdotally, not with any scientific basis, nor with an accommodation for the unique emotional condition of each human being. This is the cause of clinician stress and burnout.

This book is not about technology, equipment, regulations, policies, procedures, or medical training. There are plenty of resources for these dimensions of healthcare readily available. This is about personal performance. **This is a personal endeavor.**

This book brings together decades of clinical experience and neuroscience. We hope this book will be an invaluable asset to your becoming the best Clinician you can and want to be. We start the book with real-life stories and quickly proceed to why it is so important to master the art of learning from your past experiences. Then, we provide you with a detailed and easily understandable neuroscience framework of how the human body works; what emotions are and how they are created; and how to recognize, label, and manage them during your work, and several common situations in your day. Each chapter has both EQ and practical tips. Finally, we explore happiness and life-balance: two areas that we believe are also under trained with roots in EQ.

The goal is to not just give you tips to be a better Clinician, but to also help you understand why that tip will work for your body from a neuroscience perspective. The explicit intention is that you fully understand why these tips work so that you can make adjustments as warranted, instead of just doing things and hoping they work. When you understand the **why**, the **how** becomes much more apparent. This combination of knowledge is guaranteed to help you with your goals, and almost surely, with your personal journey of growth as well.

Throughout this book you will see numerous quotes from various backgrounds, but especially sports, used to illustrate the critical points. Multimillion dollar athletes have been incorporating *sports psychology* and emotional intelligence to make sure they are performing at the peak of their abilities for decades. In your profession, you are the *high-priced athlete*. You are performing under pressure just like an athlete. Like sports, the results in many cases are immediate – you can *see* whether what you are doing or have done is having an impact within minutes, hours, or days. The results can be enabling or disabling emotionally. Professional athletes live in this pressure-cooker world, too, but they have perfected the art and science of getting the most out of their bodies and minds. They have no choice as their careers are both lucrative and very short. These same techniques that they use could be applied to your own environment.

Essentially, two books are being provided to you: one that we wrote, and the other being written by you in the spaces provided in this book. **Thus, if you do all of the written exercises suggested, you will have a second book written by you, and for you. Either or both of these books can be read many times over during your career.**

Emotional endurance and mental strength are not just a part of healthcare, but also a part of life. It can be argued that life itself is an emotional endurance test. And this may be what makes healthcare so noble an endeavor, as you can draw parallels between work and your own life's journey. It is possible to feel many highs and lows and everything in between in one shift – a microcosm of life. Thus, investing in growing your EQ can have a profound impact on your entire life. We hope that the reader-interactive format will impact both your physical and emotional endurance to get you to perform to the best of your ability when it counts the most.

Chapter 1

"You can't control what happens to you. You can only control your response"
is a cliché we have all heard, but never really understood how to truly
personally manage. The authors lay out not only why we feel and do what
we do, but show a straightforward plan of action to improve our reaction,
overall performance, and ongoing personal mental health. These techniques
are powerful tools to help prolong careers in Emergency Medicine and
overall quality of life as clinicians.

-Michael Frye, MD, FACEP
Senior VP and Group Medical Officer
Schumacher Clinical Partners

Why Train in EQ?

So why invest in learning about Emotional Intelligence (EQ)? We
recognize that you are already strapped for time at work and the little
precious time you do have, you need for personal life. So why add
yet one more dimension to your busy life? Perhaps the best way to
establish the case for this is to review several examples of what happens
all the time in healthcare to patients and Clinicians. Below are actual
stories from physicians, nurses, and others. We had literally hundreds
to choose from, but selected just a few that underscore the fact that
emotional mishaps are virtually guaranteed to occur every day, and it
is your emotional response to them that can be the difference between
underperforming and recovering to overachieve.

Physician:

> My Dad had just recently passed after spending 1 week in
> hospice. It was my first shift back to work in the ER and it was
> hard to be there. One of my first patients was an 80-year-old
> with Parkinson's. My Dad was in his 80's and had Parkinson's.
> I was not prepared for the onslaught of emotions that overcame
> me when I walked into his room. Later in the same shift, a radio
> call came in for an elderly lady who had a terminal illness. She
> was coming from home, she was unresponsive with oxygen
> levels in the low 70's. "Family doesn't want anything done"
> was the report. Nurses nearby started to complain, "Why are
> they bringing her in if they don't want anything done? Why
> are they bringing her here if she's in hospice?" I looked at them
> and said, "Because their mom is dying in front of them and
> they don't know what to do." I waited for them to arrive and
> kept saying to myself, "Please don't let it be me. Please let one of
> my partners see her." I could have asked for help, but I didn't.
> I couldn't say anything to anyone. When the patient arrived, I
> could see she was actively dying. They put her in a room right
> in front of where I was stationed. I got up and walked in. I
> spoke with the patient's daughter and confirmed the patient's
> condition and that they didn't want any aggressive treatment.
> I told her it was ok. She did the right thing. I explained that,
> "I did this last week with my Dad." I gave her a hug and let
> her know that we would keep her Mom comfortable and make
> sure she didn't suffer. I told her I wouldn't be far if she needed
> me for anything. The patient passed away in just a few hours.
> I was in a fog for the rest of the day.

Analysis: The emotional empathy of this physician was what made his
response so different from the nurses' responses. He had just experienced
this with his own Dad and knew exactly what emotions the family
would be feeling. He used this to his advantage and responded with
compassion. **The challenge was not just medical, it was emotional.**

Nurse:

> Anna was working as charge nurse in the ER one evening. It was busy as always and some patients had been waiting. A young child had come in from an accident as a trauma patient and was critically injured. Cases like this are all-hands-on deck and all the providers were tied up trying to help. One of our chronic-regular patients began to complain. Anna explained that the doctors were tied up with a critical trauma patient and they would get to her as soon as they could. The patient began shouting, "I don't care what happens to that damn baby! Someone better come take care of me!" Anna was beside herself with anger and directed the patient back to her room. Every Clinician in the trauma heard what was said. From that moment, they all held a grudge against the chronic patient.

Analysis: Clearly what the chronic patient had said was hurtful and inappropriate. What it triggered was an emotional response from all the Clinicians. They were hurt by the callous comment. It violated their values. None of them actually talked about it because they did not know how to, but all the Clinicians showed a lack of compassion, consciously or subconsciously, towards the patient thereafter. **The challenge was not medical, it was emotional.**

Physician:

> I saw a young woman in the ER with vaginal bleeding during an early pregnancy. A common problem. During her workup, her ultrasound came back with a radiologist reading of a "blighted ovum." This means there is no embryo and she was likely having a miscarriage. I told the patient the news and did my best to give her reassurance. She later went on to have a normal pregnancy. She then wrote a long letter of complaint to my ED director saying how incompetent I was as a physician. This bothered me for a long time as I had no recourse for her to

understand that I had done everything correctly. In medicine, we can do everything right and still have a bad outcome. We are not allowed or afforded mistakes. Even in this case where me being incorrect ended with her having a baby.

Analysis: Even for the most talented and skilled Clinicians, mishaps happen. Every human body is different and you can never really know 100% how symptoms will regress or progress. The fact that it *bothered* this physician for such *a long time* means that the physician was emotionally distracted from future patients and carrying this *baggage* consciously or, for sure, subconsciously. The tragedy here is that neither the physician nor the director were emotionally trained to process this experience so that it would not be a negative experience, but rather, perhaps, a source of learning. **The challenge was not medical, it was emotional.**

Nurse:

> ➢ What stresses me most is knowing I need to be in 4 places at once. And knowing that some poor guy is going to suffer just from luck of the draw. Because he had the bad luck to come with a kidney stone at the same time as an SVT or DKA. Same goes with all level of acuity. That SVT is the most urgent patient I have, till that CPR rolls in. It always feels like the nurse's failure. Even though we logically know we are doing all we can, it is tough to look people in the eye when they demand to know why this 89-year-old had to wait in the lobby for 6 hours. Just the constant demands and reprioritizations starts to weigh on you. Not measuring up to patient's expectations has always bothered me far more than the physical or mental demands of the job.

Analysis: You can just feel the emotional toll inside this nurse. She states it herself clearly in the end what the issue is. Healthcare is a challenging environment and what makes it most challenging is not the cognitive decisions that need to be made constantly, but the emotional drain that comes with each decision. **The challenge was not medical, it was emotional.**

Physician:

> A 70-year-old woman with a history of COPD came to the ED with progressive shortness of breath. On initial exam, she was in moderate respiratory distress, tachypnic with a respiratory rate of 30, a heart rate of 110, and an oxygen saturation of 75%. She was given several breathing treatments and evaluated. After treatment, her oxygen level and work of breathing all stabilized. Ultimately, she was diagnosed with community acquired pneumonia. We talked about a course of treatment and we decided that inpatient treatment would be best. I called the admitting team and they agreed to admit the patient. About 45 minutes later, the nurse from the admitting team came and said, "Your patient in room 11 doesn't want to stay." Why would she change her mind? Why is she making a bad decision? I went back to the room and focused on her EQ at the moment. She was worried. I talked to her very calmly and reassured her that this really was important and that she should be treated in the hospital. She calmed down and thought about it and agreed to stay in the hospital. (I've seen patients be stressed for reasons you may never even think of… "I don't want to stay in the hospital, when my husband got admitted to the hospital 6 months ago he died!" or I have had patients give a *reason* that is likely more of a mental justification because of their negative emotional state, "I can't stay in the hospital! Who will feed my dog!").

Analysis: Once admitted, using logic and rational thought, emotions took over resulting in anxiety. This happens all the time as patients and their families begin to take in the new environment of a hospital room. The physician here recognized that it was not logic or medicine that was needed, but a heavy dose of compassion. **The challenge was not medical, it was emotional.**

Physician:

> A healthy 24-year-old male presented with complaints of abdominal pain. He was confrontational and verbally abusive since the moment he arrived. You treated him with doses of pain medication while you completed his workup. He still complained to the nurse swearing, "I need more f&#$ing medicine." His CT shows an acute appendicitis. You contacted the surgeon, who came to see the patient. The patient continued to rant and rave… "this is bull@#$t, you aren't treating me, I'm not f&#$ing staying." The surgeon gets agitated because of the patient's attitude, tells him that he has an acute appendicitis and needs surgery or it would likely rupture causing him to get very sick and could kill him. "I'm not staying!" "OK Fine! You can sign out against medical advice!" The patient signs out and is admitted to another hospital 12 hours later with a ruptured appendicitis.

Analysis: It is emotionally draining as a Clinician to see a patient make an illogical decision because of poor emotional control. Some Clinicians liken it to being a parent and watching your child ignore your sage advice. But this story brings into play whether changing the patient's emotions first would have resulted in his better acceptance of rational logic? We believe so. **The challenge was not medical, it was emotional.**

Physician:

> After 14 years of marriage, I came home one day to a surprise. My spouse sent the kids away and told me she wanted a divorce. She had expressed her unhappiness to me for years, but I was too tired and emotionally spent when I came back from the hospital each day. I just wanted dinner and a glass of wine and sleep. I did not know how much damage I had done to my family by being emotionally drained. I really did not

know until about six months after our divorce when I made time to attend kids' activities and my daughter came to me and said, "You never came to my games when you were married to Mom." It is easy to abdicate parental and spousal responsibility when you can justify it by saying, "I save lives every day." I've been in therapy now for 2 years unpacking how I could have become so blind emotionally. I now tell my story to all young docs and tell them not to make my mistake.

Analysis: Emotional illiteracy is not an option for Clinicians. There is a cost to this. It can be a dissatisfied patient, a wrong diagnosis, or a broken personal life. **The challenge was not medical, it was emotional.**

Senior Executive:

> ➤ As a senior executive of a large healthcare system, I am constantly amazed at how our executive team operates. We spend 90% of our time with some form of drama with each other or with physicians. Everyone seems to be in self-serving mode. A department head wants this, that, or the other. Our COO doesn't get along with our CFO, and their distrust is impacting our effectiveness. The CEO does not want to deal with it because he needs them both, because different docs are aligned with each one. It's like high school some days.

Analysis: This is not unique to healthcare, but what is unique is the matrix hierarchy. Some departments and physicians have more *power* than a CEO and that makes for a complex dynamic to lead effectively. These common issues are rarely logical. They are emotional and take their toll on overall care that institutions can provide by being too slow to react to make necessary changes. **The challenge was not medical, it was emotional.**

CIO:

> We bought a new system. Took us almost two years to implement. The physicians want me fired because it does not do everything they want. They say it keeps them from patient time. Nurses say it's too much on top of what they already do and prefer the paper world. I asked them why they did not tell us exactly what they wanted during dozens of design sessions which they missed or sent a replacement to. They said they were too busy. We have a culture that is too busy to make life better and prefers an archaic infrastructure just because they know it better, not because it is better and even though it takes them much longer. How can we change healthcare when Clinicians are not interested in changing? I'm not a psychologist – I'm a CIO. I will build whatever you want, but you have to be at the table and work with me.

Analysis: The role of emotions outside, the patient room that impacts the patient experience has largely been forgotten in the healthcare transformation conversation. New technologies and equipment are oversold, and under-deliver in many cases. The *culture* of any organization is the magic glue. Ask Disney or any other high performing culture. Consistent great results do not happen by accident. They happen because almost everyone shares a service-culture, which inherently means everyone serves everyone and will do their best to make constant changes to serve each other and patients (customers) better. **The challenge was not medical, it was emotional.**

Clearly, there are hundreds more of these kinds of stories that can be shared. Sports are a great microcosm of human performance. Professional athletes make a living counting on themselves to perform at a high level when it matters most. They get paid accordingly. Just like professional athletes, Clinicians also have a *game-time*. Depending on your area of practice, your game may require different amounts of cognitive ability or critical decision making, technical expertise and proficiency, or skill in person to person communication. Regardless of where your practice falls on this spectrum, the greatest influence on your performance will be your emotional state. **Clinicians' *game-time* is when a patient shows up.** They, too, have to perform at their absolute best regardless of what happened to the patient before or to the next patient. It is worth looking at sports and the role emotions play in performance there.

Sports

Athletes from all sports experience similar challenges. What must be noted in sports and athletes is that the common thread is how all athletes are, first, human beings built with the same physiology and neuroscience, and exhibiting the same emotional responses as Clinicians.

> ➤ In the 2016 Masters, Jordan Spieth was attempting to become the fourth player in history to win back to back tournaments, as well as his 3rd major championship. During the final round, Spieth made four consecutive birdies from holes 6-9 to open up a five-shot lead with nine holes to play. After playing his most solid nine holes of the tournament, Spieth later said that he started the back nine just trying to make pars to protect his lead. He began to hit poor shot after poor shot and made two bogeys in a row before hitting his tee shot in the water on number 12. After taking his drop, he proceeded to chunk his third shot into the water again and made a quadruple bogey. He ultimately lost the tournament by three shots. When later asked what his thinking was during those shots in the water, he said, "I don't know what I was thinking. It was a tough 30 minutes that I hope I never experience again."

Analysis: "Not being able to think clearly" is the sure sign that emotions have taken over, not that you cannot think. Managing emotions well is determined by how quickly you can think clearly again after a bad shot. **The challenge was not physical, it was emotional.**

➢ A basketball player practices free throws thousands of times and makes all of them, yet something is different when the free throw has to be made with one second to go and the game is on the line. What is different? Is it the size of the basketball? The size of the rim? The distance to the basket? Did the basketball player suddenly lose weight or get shorter or lose 20 IQ points? No, of course not. What is different is the pressure of the situation – the emotions of the situation. This is not physical, it is emotional.

➢ At an Ironman event, a pro athlete was leading the race until about mile 16 of the run when another pro athlete passed him. He had led the entire race and was shocked to get caught. So disheartened by this, he decided to try to keep up with the new leader and go faster than he knew he could. Intellectually, he knew that he could not keep up the faster pace this late in the race but chose to ignore this, and push himself even harder. By mile 22, he was spent and instead of a certain 2nd place finish, he ended up 12th. After the race, he was visibly upset. He just could not understand why he reacted the way he did when he got passed, why he abandoned his race strategy and how he let his emotions at the time he got passed cause him to ignore his training, and instead adopt a totally unrealistic running pace. He clearly underperformed and it had little to do with his physical skills.

➢ A NASCAR driver and his crew chief tell that the race is called and raced differently in the first 200 laps versus the last 50 laps. The difference between the winner and the next 10 drivers is literally seconds, so the last 50 laps are critical for finishing position. But the track is the same as it was in the first 200 laps. What is different is the pressure of those last laps where critical decisions are made. Those last laps are no longer about cars, but all about the decisions the driver and crew chief make. It is not about the equipment, but the emotions of the situation.

➤ A professional tennis player says the difference between the first four sets and the fifth set is just one thing: mental strength. She says it almost ceases to be about tennis, and whoever can remain calm in the moment of pressure and execute the shots they know they have hit thousands of times before in the fifth set almost always wins. What is the difference between the sets? What is different is the pressure of the situation – the emotions of the situation.

➤ The New York Knicks had a 105-99 lead with just 18.7 seconds left before Indiana Pacers' guard, Reggie Miller, sent them falling into one of the most stunning end-game collapses in NBA history by scoring eight points in nine mind-blowing seconds. Miller began by hitting a 3-pointer. Then he stole the ensuing inbounds pass and dashed back out to the 3-point line, where he wheeled and drained another 3 to tie the game at 105. "We were shell-shocked, we were numb," Knicks forward, Anthony Mason, remembered years later. "We became totally disoriented." The Knicks still had a few more chances to win, but John Starks missed two free throws and Knicks center, Patrick Ewing, missed a 10-footer before Miller was fouled on the rebound. He made both free throws to give the Pacers a shocking 107-105 win, and then he ran off the Madison Square Garden floor yelling, "Choke artists!" The Pacers went on to win the series in seven games.
- *Johnette Howard*

Terms like "shell-shocked" and "disoriented" used by the Knicks and so many other athletes in all sports to describe how they felt are lay terms, in effect conceding that 'something' happened to them that they cannot explain. For any athlete, there should be no part of your performance that you should not be prepared for, much less not be able to explain. The same case should be made for Clinicians – there should be no situation that you are not prepared to deal with medically and emotionally.

It should be noted that there is a fundamental difference between these kinds of stories of underperformance and others where athletes underperform because of physical reasons. If you have a strained back, it is going to be tough to perform anything athletically no matter how much emotional strength you have. When something irreparable happens to your body, no amount of EQ can compensate for that. Similarly, if you do not have the skill to do something in training, then no amount of mental strength can create that skill on the fly. You simply can't **will** yourself to do emotional strength. Clinicians are no different. If you do not have EQ skills, you will leave to chance that portion of your test when in matters most – under stress, during your shift, in front of a patient who needs you to be at your complete best.

As a neuro-sports psychologist, Dr. Justice found that disappointment and frustration does not come from failing to execute on something never done before. It comes from **the true definition of underperformance which is the inability to execute on the very things you have done many times before, but not when in matters most: during game-time**. It is the examples given above that are much harder to swallow because you feel it was something *mental* and the root cause of your poor reaction is still inexplicably a mystery to you. In these underperforming situations, you feel like you *lost* control and let something derail you. You feel like you beat yourself. This is where EQ can make a tremendous difference.

"What separates great players from the good ones is not so much ability as brain power and emotional equilibrium." -Arnold Palmer

So Why Train EQ?

As described earlier, healthcare is littered with such stories of emotional illiteracy. The consequences in sports are being defeated with a loss or less money. The consequences in healthcare are much graver to both the patient experience and the personal emotional experience of Clinicians and healthcare administrators.

If Clinicians are able to first have literacy over emotions, and skills to manage them, then they can maintain composure, access their medical training memories, and simply perform as they have trained. Subsequently, their chances of being successful go up significantly. This is obvious. How to do it is not so obvious. ***This is why we train in EQ.*** We prepare ourselves to stay focused and positive in the midst of mishaps and distractions so that we can perform our best - be it in sports or in the arena of patient care.

This fundamental shift in reframing how you view and do your job - with emotional competence - is the first step in building your EQ.

We define emotional strength as the amount of time it takes to convert a negative thought (stimuli) to a positive one.

It is impossible to predict what is going to go wrong and when it will happen, but suffice it to say, in all likelihood something will happen that will cause anxiety during your day at the hospital or clinic. This we can all agree on. And if you concede this, then, in order to perform at your best in front of every patient, you must prepare to manage your emotions and thoughts. A plan that incorporates EQ training will help you manage the unpredictable, but certain-to-occur, anxiety-inducing experiences and your responses to them. As noted in the introduction, if you are going to spend your life doing something so noble and rewarding, why not spend just a few minutes a day to grow your EQ and remain positive and focused in the throes of situations that are beyond your control? No one wishes for chaos of any kind, but **a positive recovery from a bad situation can actually be incredibly motivating and powerful to spur you on to an even better performance.**

"Life is 10% what happens to you and 90% how you react to it." -Charles R. Swindoll

Please take a few moments to write down in your own words an experience where you underperformed during a shift with a patient or co-worker, similar to the stories shared earlier in this chapter. In subsequent chapters, as tips are shared, you will be asked to come back to this story and personalize your learning. By writing down your own personal experiences, your own emotions and presence in the experience will make the learning, and subsequent growth, a much richer endeavor. As you write your story, try to describe yourself emotionally, mentally, and physically, as well as describe the situation you were in as graphically as you can.

Note that a mishap is not just a situation where something has gone terribly wrong, like the stories described earlier, but mishaps can be anything where you have lost your focus and as a result, deviated from your capabilities and underperformed.

Exercise: My Personal Story of Under-Performing

| **Top 3 Ideas** |
| *I learned from this chapter* |
| 1. |
| 2. |
| 3. |
| |
| **3 Action Steps** |
| *I will take immediately to incorporate the above learning into my day* |
| 1. |
| 2. |
| 3. |

Chapter Summary

1. Emotions play a major role in all your interactions and performances as a Clinician.
2. Professional sports and athletes offer a good reference framework to perform at high levels under pressure.
3. When mishaps happen, our emotions are tested. This emotional test is what most Clinicians are undertrained in, yet, could be a game-changer.
4. When your emotional reaction to a situation is poor, your decision-making is compromised and you underperform.
5. The cumulative effect of unresolved emotional stress results in decreased performance, compassion fatigue, and Clinician burnout.

Chapter 2

"It is very important to understand that emotional intelligence is not the opposite of intelligence, it is not the triumph of heart over head--it is the unique intersection of both." -David Caruso

Neuroscience of a Clinician

It is critical that you understand how your body works physiologically. Your body is the ultimate equipment in your work. If you can shell out tens of thousands, or hundreds of thousands of dollars on a medical education, and spend years specializing in your field, then consider spending quality time on understanding your body as a piece of equipment that you need to appreciate with the same amount of passion and detail. Unlike your *stethoscope* or whatever tool you use, however, your body (emotions and thoughts) is constantly changing, which makes understanding it even more important. Imagine using machines that changed constantly and only gave good data if and when they *felt* good that day? That would be crazy and a recipe for disaster. Yet, that is exactly what is happening to your emotions after each experience – they are constantly changing. **The most important equipment that you use in every patient experience, your body and mind, is constantly changing!**

When we coach Clinicians, one of the first questions we ask them is to describe their favorite piece of equipment to us. If it is a machine, the Clinician will describe in infinite detail all the information that the machine provides that takes most of the guess work from the past out, allowing them to make much better decisions for the Clinician. Maybe it is a cat scan or MRI or whatever. After the detailed description, we pause and then ask for a description of his or her brain. We get the same reaction you just had. "Huh?"

If all the decisions are made in only one part of your body — and that's your brain — then of all the tools and skills to master, knowing your brain and how it works is the singular most important skill all Clinicians, healthcare support staff, and administrators alike, should invest in.

How many decisions do you have to make with each patient experience? Please take a few moments to do the following exercise.

Exercise: Decisions made in one patient experience

Make a list of most common cognitive decisions you have to make in just one patient experience.

1._____

2._____

3._____

4._____

5._____

6._____

7._____

8._____

9._____

10._____

There are probably another 10 you can easily come up with. So, as you can see, there are a ton of decisions to be made in just one patient experience and hundreds more during the day. And they are all made in and by only one part of your body: your brain. Understanding how your brain functions is fundamental.

Superior Performance

The ultimate goal for you as a Clinician is to perform at your best when the patient is in front of you, when it matters most. Not on your drive home afterwards and not during case reviews, but when it matters most: during *game-time* - when every decision really counts. Period. Good and timely decision-making, which only occurs in the brain is at the heart of optimal performance, where you are able to harness all your training as a Clinician and recall pertinent past experiences. Your ability to make decisions, therefore, is the centerpiece to optimal performance, since without it, you are guaranteed to underperform.

This begins the understanding of how decisions are made. There is a neurological sequence with how all decisions are made. Let us start with the end result and work backwards.

As shown below, superior performance is the end game with good decision-making at the center of it.

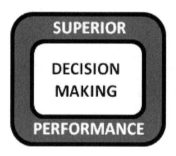

Figure 1. Superior Performance

Competency

The way that you know you are making good decisions during a patient visit or key event is directly related to your ability to execute your training and experience, or competencies. Competencies or skills are the things we know how to do because of how we have trained. This would include taking a patient history, performing a physical exam, and formulating a care plan or plan of action. This would also include procedural skills like a wound repair, placing a central line, reducing a fracture, or an operative procedure. This also includes interpreting diagnostic tests: reading an EKG, a blood gas, or CT scan. They are specific skills and abilities, such as the medical training of your discipline. Clinicians have invested an enormous amount of time here. In other words, good training plays a big part in decision-making and subsequent performance. But most of you already know this.

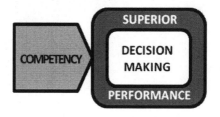

Figure 2. Competency

Behavior

Preceding our competencies and skills, are our behaviors. See below for the sequence of understanding how good decisions are made.

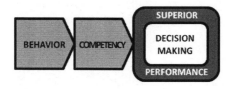

Figure 3. Behavior

Behaviors are essentially the framework of how we show our thoughts and emotions. Showing the emotion of happiness by smiling or the emotion of anger by yelling are the behaviors we all know well. All of us know people who have mastered specific competencies (skills) in life, but some inadequate or inappropriate behaviors have diluted their competencies, which in turn, compromises their ability to perform at high levels. So these people, although full of skill/talent, let their innate talent go to waste because of poor behavior. In healthcare, when things do go wrong, it is the responsive behavior that everyone sees.

Behavior is a response. Make no mistake about it. It is a response (not cause) to your brain's interpretation of an experience.

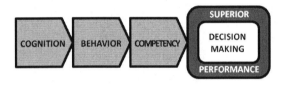

Figure 4. Cognition & Behavior

Cognition

Cognition precedes behavior. Slightly oversimplifying this concept, cognition refers to one's intellectual capacities, thoughts, knowledge, and memories. This is the rational part of our brain. In effect, it is our ability to take data points, weave them together in some cogent manner, and reach a conclusion that dictates (consciously or subconsciously) what behavior to exhibit. This includes the sum total of your medical knowledge. If your knowledge base is lacking, then, regardless of your behavior or skills, you are going to under-perform. If your thinking leads to the wrong conclusion, the rest of the steps in the sequence to good decision-making get compromised, no matter how competent (skilled) you are.

You can now begin to see all the pieces of decision-making in a sequence, where each preceding dimension can trump the proceeding dimension.

"Experience is not what happens to you--it's how you interpret what happens to you." -Aldous Huxley

Emotional Intelligence (EQ)

What finally precedes cognition in this physiological sequence to decision-making (high performance) is your Emotional Intelligence (EQ). This key area has likely been neglected, and if so, will, to some extent, sabotage all the years of hard work.

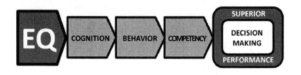

Figure 5. Emotional Intelligence (EQ)

What you see above is the neurological sequence in the brain of human beings for all decision-making, whether it is in healthcare or in day-to-day life. Emotions are the first neurological response by your body, the equipment. Your physical body is an equipment that you want to manipulate correctly for a required decision. **Everything in your body and brain is dictated first by your emotions.** Emotions lead to thinking, which leads to behavior, which is the uniform you wear as you perform your skills. You can see how easily it is for your skills to be compromised, especially in the heat of the moment as they are so farther down the sequence. Skills stand no chance against the power of your emotions and how your brain is interpreting stimuli, especially in real time (*game-time*) when everything seemingly is at stake, and happening at warp speed.

Our five senses aggressively and constantly send signals to the prefrontal lobes of the brain located in our forehead area. This is the *port of entry* of all stimuli. Everything we see, hear, feel, touch, and smell gets sent here for primarily one purpose: to assign a threat rating to that experience. Happening in microseconds, the higher the threat level, the more the secretion of powerful hormones like cortisol (fear), which can cause high states of anxiety. The lower the threat level, the smoother the transition into the subsequent steps of the diagram above, allowing you to think clearly, behave appropriately, and ultimately perform to your ability.

"Of all the hazards, fear is the worst." -Sam Snead

Neuroscience of "Pressure"

The terms anxiety, nerves, pressure, disoriented, stress, heat-of-battle/moment, choking, being-in-the-zone, and the like, are used not only in all sports, but also everyday life when performing any function that can be evaluated. Let us dig deeper into understanding our body, the equipment, in the context of these terms.

Our brain is the only place where all our cognitive functions reside. Cognitive functions include our long-term, short-term, and working memory. Put simply, the brain is ***both*** our filing cabinet and command center to make decisions. For example, if you have just learned how to use a new EMR system, that learning sits in your brain, not in your hands or arms. There is no such thing as muscle memory. Muscles do not have any memory cells or neuropathic abilities. You can train your muscles and body parts new motor skills, but in terms of the command to execute those new skills, that comes from the brain. A person in a coma, whose body is perfectly normal, is unable to perform any physical activity because the command center, the brain, is disabled. **Everything you know and have learned is stored in the brain.** The same brain that you are using for a patient encounter is also where all of your life's experiences are stored. This is a key point in the context of underperforming, as Clinicians often wonder after an unsatisfactory patient experience why they made poor decisions, or say "in hindsight" they may have made better decisions and behaved differently with a patient.

From the command center, the brain, all orders are sent to different parts of the body. The body itself cannot do anything without the brain. The brain sends all its instructions through the spinal cord. In other words, the spinal cord is like a bundle of cables for that critical information from memory banks to be sent to parts of your body. Now, as shown in the next image, conveniently located between the spinal cord and the brain — between the command center and cables — is the amygdala.

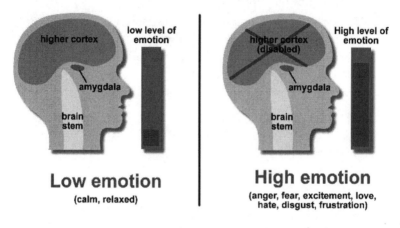

Figure 6. Impact of Emotions

The Instinctive Emotional Response

The amygdala is a gland that secretes hormones in your body, as noted earlier. It is situated there because its job is to respond according to the directions of the prefrontal lobes – the threat center. The prefrontal lobes sit in your forehead area. Microseconds of sensing a potential threat, the amygdala (and other glands) releases hormones in your body that either partially or entirely disables your brain. This disabling of cognitive functions enables your body to respond quickly and instinctively to that danger. This is essentially a safety mechanism, which is triggered as a reaction to every threat, regardless of whether the danger is perceived or real. *Our bodies have spent thousands of years morphing into this state so that we can perform our primary function: recognize danger and react to survive.* This is no different than most other living organisms. Although there are some universal physical dangers, such as someone pointing a gun at you, most emotional threats have no standards. It is different for everyone and based entirely on one's past experiences, memory banks, and mostly, from childhood or previous failures.

For example, if you are crossing a road and you see a car coming at you from the corner of your eye, you would — without thinking — instinctively jump or run to get the heck out of the way. You would not think about it; you would not analyze, "I wonder how fast the car is going. What are my options here?" If you did that — if you used the cognitive functions of your brain — you would not be able to respond fast enough and you would be hit. Therefore, the brain has to be disabled quickly for you to instinctively jump out of the way of the car.

Similarly, because it is the same brain, cognitive functions are disabled when Clinicians get into situations that they perceive as danger, such as going to meet your boss or having a patient suddenly collapse, knowing that all of a sudden you have gone from making inconsequential decisions (perhaps in the breakroom) to a very consequential situation. The physiological response in the body in critical situations is virtually identical to that of a car coming at you. In other words, the amygdala does not make the distinction between the threat of a car coming at you and the threat of the consequences of poor decisions made in front of a patient where the consequences are very real. They are both threats, yet one is physical and the other is emotional.

"We are all faced with a series of great opportunities brilliantly disguised as impossible situations." -Charles R. Swindoll

Look at the body's physiological automatic and instinctive response to anything perceived as a negative experience, depicted in Figure 7. In this state, just look at the impact of negative emotions on the physical body, the same body that you need to use around a patient. No athlete can perform at his/her best in this state and neither can a Clinician.

This is akin to being physically injured! In every patient experience, as already discussed, a Clinician is guaranteed to be in this state. And even if something does not go wrong, body fatigue, peer pressure, and life pressure, all force the amygdala to do its instinctive job.

This physiological state leads to a *high alert state,* where the brain is operating in *lock down mode* similar to the scenario of the speeding car approaching. The following consequences apply in this state:

- Have decreased cognitive performance.
- Have less oxygen available for critical brain functions.
- Tend to over generalize.
- Respond with defensive action.
- Perceive small stressors as worse than they actually are.
- Are easily aggravated.
- Recollection of past negative experiences.
- Will struggle to get along with others.
- Cannot perform at your best.

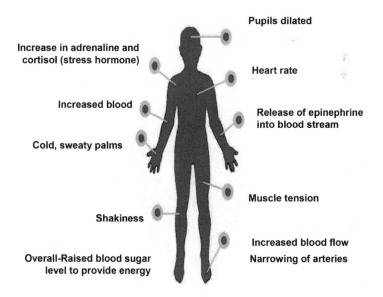

Figure 7. The Body's Auto-Responsive Physiology

This state leads to those negative monologues – where we doubt our training, question our will, and recall past negative situations unintentionally. At that point, access to our rational ability and skill memory has been disabled and we are in the instinctive fight-or-flight mode. Again, no Clinician can perform at his/her best in this state. He/she simply is hijacked by his/her own body in the most natural and instinctive of ways. It is a virtual guarantee that every Clinician will be in this state several times during a day. The question then becomes of how to manage this state, and this is where emotional intelligence (EQ) comes in.

"It's this simple: If I never try anything, I never learn anything. If I never take a risk, I stay where I am." -Hugh Prather

Negative Monologues

There is arguably no greater threat to a Clinician than his or her own negative monologue. We all have them, not just in our jobs, but also in our lives. You know the ones where you talk to yourself about all the reasons why you cannot or should not do something, where you recall the worse memories, and seriously doubt your ability to perform. There is no Clinician or human being who actively pursues a negative monologue. They happen without choice, and very often at the most inopportune of times.

Conversely, athletes and Clinicians often say that when they are at their best, in the proverbial zone, that there is no such negative monologue. In fact, the calm state is almost euphoric as though everything is exactly how it should be and they are performing magic.

In healthcare, which is very much like an endurance sport of many hours, you are certain to have both types of dialogues (positive and negative). We will discuss at length how to manage your emotions and these dialogues; but first, it is important to understand how the negative ones, more harmful to your performance, are created.

Let us say you had 10 experiences yesterday and nine of them were spectacular ones – very positive – but one of them was negative. For example, the negative one may have been you accidentally touching a hot stove and slightly burning your hand while making coffee. Today, the day after, which experience do you think you will be remembering more? If you answered honestly, then it would be the negative one, not the other nine great positive ones. Why? Once again, our physiological design and construction from thousands of years takes center stage. Our brain has a specific place in the back of our skull where, in fact, negative memories are stored. When we have negative experiences in life, whether traumatic ones or like the slight hand burn, the brain needs to store them so that they can easily be retrieved. You NEED to remember the burned hand more than the nine positive experiences because the burned hand plays a larger role in your survival than your positive experiences. You need to remember to be careful next time you are near a hot stove.

In this manner, almost all of our life's negative experiences are not only permanently stored, but they are in fact the ones that are first retrieved if the prefrontal lobes (Threat Center) label a current experience as a negative one (one with potential threat). So as the amygdala disables the brain in high anxiety situations after getting word from the prefrontal lobes, your cognitive functions (making decisions, remembering how to do routine skills) are further limited to those negative memories and, thus, the negative monologues. A Clinician, who was nervous going to an already-upset patient's room, recalls that he remembered what had happened just the day before in a similar situation as the latter was not a positive experience. Even though it was a completely different day and different patient (nor in any way related to the current patient), given that his brain was on alert, he then recalled his own negative memory. This is all happening because our brain is searching for context for the current threat alert.

It is, therefore, very important for a Clinician to take inventory of those past negative experiences so that he or she is, at a bare minimum, aware of what they are and can anticipate the nature of the negative monologues when they occur. In this book, you will learn how to do this as well as how to proactively induce positive monologues during your day; but more importantly, during those unpredictable critical situations.

Sometimes these experiences are easier to recognize. A situation triggers an acute negative response in you. These triggers can be completely different for each Clinician. For one person it may be an irate patient or family member; for another, it might be a sick kid. While for someone else it might be the manipulative drug seeking patient. Other times the stressors are smaller and cumulative. It could simply be the mounting pressures of the day and dealing with the unexpected bumps in the road. However, the end result is the same. You are in a heightened state of stress and your brain is responding to threats. Your performance suffers.

Exercise: Your Negative Memory Bank

Make a list of the experiences of your life that you feel are possibly stored in your negative memory bank.

1._____

2._____

3._____

4._____

5._____

"Live as if you were to die tomorrow. Learn as if you were to live forever." -Mahatma Gandhi

Exercise: Your Negative Monologues

Make a list of most common negative monologues you typically have with yourself after a bad experience.

1._____

2._____

3._____

4._____

5._____

Exercise: Your Positive Monologues

Make a list of the most common positive monologues you have with yourself (when you are in a zone).

1._____

2._____

3._____

4._____

5._____

Top 3 Ideas		
I learned from this chapter		
1.		
2.		
3.		
3 Action Steps		
I will take immediately to incorporate the above learning into my work and personal life		
1.		
2.		
3.		

Chapter Summary

1. Your goal needs to be to perform at your best during the patient experience. This means making good decisions.
2. The physiological sequence of making good decisions starts with our emotions, not our skills or thinking. Therefore, understanding emotions is critical to optimal performance.
3. All our medical training and skills are stored in our brain, and in no other part of our body. The brain can be shut off as an instinctive survival response to any danger, perceived or real. When the brain is disabled, then poor decisions are made.

Chapter 3

I worked 18 years in a busy L&D in a large city. When faced with the comment, "Oh it must be so nice to work in such a happy place and just play with babies all day!" I often had to bite my tongue. Yes, while L&D is generally happy, when things go bad - they go really bad. Unfortunately, these situations are not that uncommon. I admit I got burned out with the low staffing numbers, high patient acuity level; even our teamwork and communication were suffering. I left a job that I had once loved because I just couldn't handle the emotional stress anymore. While I love working in Nursing Education, Healthcare EQ would have been a lifesaver for me in those last 5 years of my career in L&D. I wish this resource was available then. I not only love the content in the book, but I love that I am actively participating in my learning by reflecting on my own experiences and brainstorming future techniques! I plan on working some part-time hours again in L&D and look very forward to utilizing the techniques to control the emotional temperature of myself and my colleagues. The helpful strategies in this book have proven useful in my personal life as well!

-Sarah Scibetta, RN

Changing Your Emotional Temperature

How to Increase your EQ

The first step in increasing your EQ is to learn to take your emotional temperature. Imagine an old mercury thermometer – the kind you stick in your mouth. Imagine there are only three recordings it can give you – GREEN, YELLOW, and RED – similar to that of a traffic light.

31

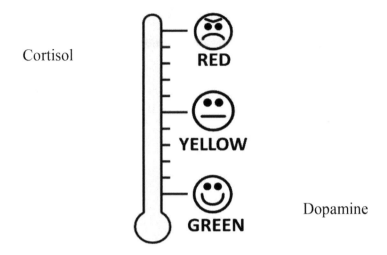

Figure 8. Emotional Thermometer

GREEN indicates that you are comfortable, happy, stress-free, can think clearly, and perform well. Now that you understand the neuroscience behind GREEN, you will note that the prefrontal lobes have sent a low threat level signal to the amygdala while in this state. This essentially means your brain, where all of the memories of your training and strategy are stored, can easily retrieve skills, memories, and make good decisions — the center piece of your performing at your best. It also means that the negative memories do not have to be accessed, which enhances your chances of being in a zone, since only positive monologues occur here. GREEN is a good temperature reading. You can learn how to give yourself an accurate reading by referring to the diagram above showing the body's state when RED. When GREEN, you will naturally feel relaxed, you will feel like all your senses are alert, you will naturally have positive monologues and recall positive experiences, you will remember all of your focal thoughts in all the parts of your training and discipline, and you will feel like nothing can throw you off your game.

YELLOW temperature reading indicates that you are a little stressed and anxious. Something has gone wrong in the day, but it is not fatal.

Perhaps your child was ill, or a physician was insensitive to you, or a nurse forgot to get you the information you needed – the list goes on and on of things that can go wrong and take us off "GREEN" to "YELLOW". You are not in GREEN for sure because everything just described for that is not happening, but you are also not in RED where the consequences are very serious. In YELLOW, negative dialogues are occurring, but you are able to recollect some positive ones too. It is an internal battle. Most of your day may feel like this.

RED is when you are implicitly or explicitly out of control, filled with anger and rage, or disappointment and frustration. You are filled with negative monologues, even being abusive to yourself and perhaps others around you, such as your co-workers or patients. You are looking to blame someone, instead of finding a solution. You are frustrated that you cannot think clearly or remember much. This happens when the perceived threat is interpreted in your brain as fatal – at this point, you feel failure of some sort is imminent and very likely.

"When you're playing poorly, you start thinking too much. That's when you confuse yourself." -Greg Norman

This is a new language you are now learning to use in healthcare – GREEN, YELLOW, and RED. Identifying how your body is at any given point of the day. You can see now why it is so important to know your EQ temperature during your shift. The good news is that taking your emotional temperature is not something you can only practice at work. Remember how all decisions are made, not just healthcare ones? Everything starts with emotions, in and out of healthcare. So, no matter where you are or what you are doing, every three hours of a normal day, starting today, take your emotional temperature and give yourself a color reading. Are you GREEN, YELLOW, or RED? After about a week of this, start to do it more often, perhaps every hour and then start to do it during your shift. We recommend taking your EQ temperature before every patient experience knowing that if you are not GREEN, you are going to underperform.

This simple language, GREEN, YELLOW, and RED, is a powerful tool in understanding your emotions, which is the ultimate trump card in the decision-making process. Consider this statement:

The quarterback stepped back and threw a long pass, which the wide receiver caught. He stayed in bounds, missed several tackles, and dove into the end zone for a touchdown.

If you are an American, chances are that you completely understand that this is about a play in the game of football. There are some terms used here that are used nowhere else that help you understand the game of football. Terms like quarterback, long pass, wide receiver, in bounds, tackles, end zone, and touch down.

Similarly, without having a language to understand emotional temperature and emotions, it is virtually impossible to decipher what is happening emotionally. Recall from Chapter 1, the challenge was not medical, it was emotional. Consider the power of everyone in your unit having the same emotional language. Most of us, neither in formal schools nor in personal lives, have ever been taught an emotional language.

As stated earlier, ***the most difficult patient experience is the one right after a bad one.*** You know why now. After a bad one, you are assured, without any active provocation from yourself, to retrieve other negative memories, disable your brain, and compromise your decision-making ability. You are either YELLOW or RED after a bad experience. For this reason, the proceeding experience is the most difficult one because you are in an internal war now between your will and your instinctive biological state. Your body, your equipment has changed. Getting your body out of YELLOW or RED and back to GREEN is EQ. How to win this before you get to the next experience is described in detail later.

You must become a master at taking your own temperature. Clearly, if you are GREEN, then nothing needs to be done mentally or emotionally. Just keep going and maintain your focus. But if you are

YELLOW or RED, then something has to happen to get you back to GREEN as fast as possible. Research has shown that it is rare to go from GREEN directly to RED unless something very dramatic happens. Usually, we progress slowly into YELLOW without being aware of it, and stay in YELLOW for a while, at which point, nothing dramatic is required to elevate to RED since you are essentially a fuse just waiting to be lit. This is another common mistake many Clinicians make. They do not do enough when in YELLOW to get back to GREEN and often think they are mentally strong to go from RED directly back to GREEN. This can be done, but it is much harder.

Once you have learned how to take your EQ temperature, then, and only then, can you know how to regulate yourself back to GREEN. The things you would do to go from YELLOW back to GREEN are very different from the things you would do to go from RED back to GREEN. Not every mishap is a RED. Having a co-worker yell at you is very different from having a patient yell at you – emotionally.

To state the obvious, the goal is to stay in GREEN as much as possible. Note that this is an emotional state. Chapters 4 through 8 discuss very specific mishap situations — emotional and mental — to help with typical scenarios in healthcare. In this chapter, by establishing these GREEN, YELLOW, and RED standards, you now have a language you can use with your peers and family to help you prepare in a customized manner.

Changing your Emotional Temperature: GREEN TO GREEN

Our five senses are the only connection our body, the equipment, has with ever-changing stimuli. As you take your EQ temperature during any given day prior to every patient experience, and you are GREEN, then the goal is to stay GREEN proactively. When already in GREEN, the best way to stay in GREEN is to actively overuse your five senses. This is called macro and micro FOCUS, and discussed in further detail in Chapter 4.

You would be using your eyes, for example, to focus on the smallest detail of whatever is in front of you. It might be a patient's face or hands, or trees and clouds outside, or specific colors on flowers. For FEEL, you would not just be feeling for what you are holding, but the air around you in every room and even the air coming in and out of your lungs. Or even feel the energy transfer from your arms and legs as you walk up and down the floor, or the sense of your hands on gripping a pen or equipment. For SOUND, it would not be just listening for voices, but other sounds you normally would ignore, such as perhaps the humming and beeping noises of equipment on the clinic floor. For TASTE, it can be allowing a sip of water or drink to sit in your mouth for a few seconds longer than normal or doing the same thing with any food.

Actively engaging the senses is a powerful technique to stay in the proverbial present, and to keep your self-awareness at a high state of alert. Think about it – if you are this focused and you notice that suddenly, for whatever reason you are not, then you know your emotional temperature has changed. Something has caused you to lose focus. It is hard to know you have lost focus if you never had it in the first place. We discuss focus in greater detail and how to use it in both training and *game-time* situations in Chapter 4. For now, learn to appreciate your five senses as a critical tool set in the equipment of your body.

"The successful warrior is the average man, with laser-like focus." -Bruce Lee

Changing your Emotional Temperature: YELLOW TO GREEN

The absolute first thing to do when you take your EQ temperature and you are in YELLOW is to breathe. This might surprise you since you are probably thinking that you are always breathing – what is up with that? No. Change your breathing. Take a count (cadence) of how long it takes you to breathe in, and take another count of how long it takes you to breathe out in the same normal breath. For most people, this normal breathing count is anywhere from 2-5 counts breathing in, and

2-5 counts breathing out. Practice right now and increase your breath count in to average about 25 and your breath count out to average about 25 also. You can do this by simply taking in your breath slower and releasing your breath longer in a very controlled manner. When the body physiologically is in YELLOW, recall that one of the symptoms is increased heart rate and increased respiratory rate. A lot of oxygen is being channeled to other parts of your body in anticipation of having to *jump to avoid the car*, but it is your brain that needs the oxygen. Slowing your breath by actively counting 25 in and 25 out, will slow down your heart rate, even if just a little at first and begin to disable the amygdala and enable the brain. Recall that it is only in your brain where all your skills reside. You need your memories of skills and what-to-do list. This kind of EQ breathing allows you to use some rational thought by putting the situation that caused you to go to YELLOW into context.

ACT (Abdomen, Chest, Throat) Breathing Technique

During physical activity, and especially during a critical situation, there are essentially three levels of breathing that occur. The first is breathing at the throat (T) level – air tends not to feel like it goes anywhere deeper than your mouth. This is typically short and fast breaths where the breath-count in and out is less than 2. The second is chest (C) level, where the breaths are inhaled chest-deep, with breath-counts in and out between 2 and 10. The last is abdomen (A) level, where a long slow breath in, to the level your lungs feel like they are touching your abdomen, is followed by a long slow breath out.

During a normal day, most Clinicians are not thinking of their breath at all and allow it to be at the mercy of whatever happens. High anxiety situations also automatically trigger your body to the T level of breathing. This is instinctive and in response to the higher heart rate – which itself is a response by the body to prepare you for survival. Unlike cognitive or brain activity, breathing involves a lot of body parts and muscles and, therefore, can be controlled even after the initial burst of anxiety to T level breathing. This is the reason why it should always be the first step in managing EQ – because it is one of the easiest things to do. Though A level (abdomen) breathing is quite challenging to maintain all day long, your goal should be to always be breathing at A level during *game-time* – in times of challenging conditions. We also recommend attempting A level breathing when you are GREEN. As you are training or playing, keep track of what level of ACT (Abdomen, Chest, Throat) you are doing and know you can perform best at the A level, so adjust your breathing accordingly. Learning this is key to building EQ strength.

The next step in changing your temperature from YELLOW to GREEN is to create a YELLOW CARD. This card will change over time, and maybe even several times, over the course of a year. Let's create your personalized YELLOW card first and then we will elaborate on how to use it to change the temperature (after breathing) from YELLOW to GREEN. Answer the next five questions with just three words or less that will instantly take you back emotionally to a very specific point in time and place.

Exercise: Your Yellow Card
1. When/where was the best patient experience you have ever had?
2. When/where was the most recent compliment you received from a patient?
3. When/where was the last patient experience where you turned a negative situation into a positive outcome?
4. When/where was the best vacation you recently had?
5. When/where was the best compliment you received from your coworkers/administrators?

Transfer these questions and your responses to a yellow index card (for your pocket when working) or perhaps onto your mobile device (during off times) so that it is portable and can be with you when you need it.

Just as negative and threatening experiences have dire consequences to the chemistry of our body as explained earlier, positive experiences have the opposite effect. They can give us confidence by releasing dopamine (happy hormone), the counter hormone to cortisol (fear hormone) and inspire us to perform better. Research shows that it takes an average of five positive experiences to dilute a comparable negative experience. In other words, cortisol is more powerful than dopamine. Recall the burnt hand example from earlier versus the nine great things on that day. The problem during work, and especially during a long shift, is that we cannot predict when those positive experiences will happen, any more than we can predict when the negatives one will occur. However, we can be certain that it is very unlikely that the positive experiences will conveniently occur immediately as the negative one is happening so that they can counteract each other out. Fortunately for us, our brain does not differentiate between a current experience and a remembered previous experience. This is where the YELLOW card comes in. These five positive experiences can be induced into your physiological system to redirect the neuropathways. They are impossible to remember during the *heat* of a situation as you have so many competing thoughts and priorities, and therefore writing them down before hand is necessary. You will need this list to counteract the cause of what got you into YELLOW so you can get back to GREEN.

After your breathing, when in YELLOW, take a look at the YELLOW card you have crafted for yourself. It is critical that you have written down on a card for reading later when needed, as opposed to relying on memory. Forget how it will look like to a co-worker – at this point, your biggest enemy is not another person, it is yourself.

When working, as you read it, take just a minute to transport yourself emotionally to that great memory and remember what worked so well and what you are capable of doing. The breathing and the YELLOW card (induced positive counteracting experiences) will impact your prefrontal lobes, the *grip* of the amygdala, and allow you to do what you need to do to get back to focusing and to GREEN.

Take note that you are using both your emotions (by taking your temperature) and your thoughts first, prior to using your medical skills to get to performing at your best again – just as the sequential physiological decision-making model dictates.

If you look at some people's office spaces, you will often see a photo of someone and other meaningful trinkets. Maybe it is a picture of loved ones or a hero in their lives. Looking at them *makes them feel good*. These pictures or mementos work in the same way, and often times bring an individual's emotions back from YELLOW to GREEN. The difference is that you are proactive about them and are consciously using them everywhere you go, instead of just placing them somewhere.

Hostage negotiators use this same technique when working with criminals who have taken hostages. They know the situation is RED, the criminal is RED, and so are the hostages. Their first goal is to *emotionally diffuse* the situation to allow rational thought to have a chance. Sometimes, they will bring in the wife or child of the criminal to talk to them directly. Hearing their voices can be a very powerful dilutor of RED emotions that can allow for a safe resolution.

When in YELLOW or RED, you are your own hostage negotiator as you are being held captive emotionally and cognitively by thousands of years of design and your own negative memories.

Changing your Emotional Temperature: RED TO GREEN

When something terrible has occurred and you have taken your emotional temperature and diagnosed yourself as RED, the first step is again to immediately breathe in the same way as the process for YELLOW to GREEN. This will be a little harder, but more important, to do. Try your best to get to A Level (Abdomen) of breathing. In RED, your breathing will be very intense (T level), your heart rate very high and your vision blurred, just to a mention a few symptoms.

The process to go from RED to GREEN is similar to the YELLOW transformation. You need to create a RED card, but the content will be very different. You will still need to induce positive experiences, but they have to be of a very different and very powerful kind.

> My first Ironman race as a pro was in 2002 at Ironman Wisconsin. One reason I became a professional was that I wanted to do the Wisconsin race as that was near my hometown of Sussex. I spent the year training, going to Madison and working on the course, and was very confident going into it. I attended the press conference, which I was not invited to, but still went and listened. No one knew who I was. Listening to the pro women, I still had belief in myself and that I could win. I registered and received my lucky number 33 and thought I was all ready. During the race I had a fabulous win. I saw the top pro ahead of me and passed her on the bike with all media camera on me now! I had a phenomenal bike ride, but when I got off the bike my legs hurt so badly that I couldn't run. I ran anyway but couldn't keep up, started walking and got passed. Half way, on the sidelines I saw my daughter and mother-in-law, both in their wheelchairs, screaming for me, and thought how awful that I was feeling sorry for myself for having aching legs. They would have given anything to walk just a mile. I ran over- gave them a hug and high five, and started running again with only their faces on my mind, and won the Ironman.
>
> -Heather Gollnick
>
> 5-Time Ironman Champion

Though Heather's story above has nothing to do with healthcare, it is very powerful and clearly was incredibly effective to get her from almost not finishing at the half way mark of the run, to winning the Ironman in 2002; and underscores just how powerful emotions can be. The same applies to healthcare. You, however, may not have your daughter and mother-in-law in a wheelchair during your critical situation every day, and do not need to, to orchestrate a similar transformation in yourself during a RED state situation. You can self-induce similarly powerful experiences by completing the RED card below. The RED card, unlike the YELLOW one, rarely changes and is used in those rare RED situations we all hope not to have.

Your personalized RED Card: Answer the five questions below with just three words or less that will instantly take you back to that point in memory, time, and place.

Exercise: Your Red Card
1. What are the first names of the most important people in your life?
2. What are the first names of your best friends – the ones that will be your friends for life?
3. When/where was the place you have been happiest in your life?
4. Who is the person, dead or alive, that you aspire to be like and why?
5. What are you most proud of in your life – an accomplishment not given to you that no one can ever take from you?

The YELLOW and RED experiences are YOUR positive experiences and one of the more under-utilized assets you have. You know your brain will neurologically attract YOUR negative memories when in YELLOW or RED. It is designed to do so. Your job is to attract positive ones at the right time, after bad situations, between patients, so that you can make the best decision for the next patient, and allow your brain to do what you have trained it to do and know you are capable of doing.

Now, let's redefine emotional strength:

Emotional strength is the amount of time it takes to convert a negative thought to a positive one.

Emotional strength is the amount of time it takes to go from YELLOW to GREEN.

Emotional strength is the amount of time it takes to go from RED to GREEN.

Top 3 Ideas
I learned from this chapter
1.
2.
3.
3 Action Steps
I will take immediately to incorporate the above learning into my work and personal life
1.
2.
3.

Chapter Summary

1. Knowing your emotional temperature at all times of the day is critical to your performance. There are 3 EQ Temperature readings: GREEN, YELLOW, and RED.

2. The goal is to stay GREEN as much as possible by using the ACT Breathing Model and your five senses to focus.

3. If in YELLOW or RED, use cards (or similar approach) to induce positive experiences (dopamine) to counteract the impact of any daily negative experiences (cortisol).

4. These techniques begin to lay the foundation of being a Clinician with high EQ.

Chapter 4

As a nurse educator, I look forward to incorporating the emotional intelligence tools in my toolbox when utilizing case studies in the classroom and also during post conference. Emotional intelligence will enable novice healthcare workers to cope with the demands of growing dynamic healthcare systems, and with the high volume and acuity of patient populations. In addition, as a practicing obstetric, registered nurse, emotional intelligence will benefit me on days when a pregnancy does not have the expected outcome for the patient and her family.

-Dina Khentigan, MSN, RN, C-EFM, CPFI

Art and Science of Learning

Healthcare requires a good bit of IQ (intellectual intelligence) as cognitive functions are put to the test. Every patient can be diagnosed by asking the right questions and doing the right tests. Years of medical training and experience lead to better diagnosis and treatment. This was discussed earlier, but it is worth now making the distinction much clearer.

There are essentially three categories of skills that are tested in caregiving:

1) Medical Skills
2) Mental Skills
3) Emotional Skills

Medical skills are obvious: your experience and training in your specialty allow you to do your job. As stated earlier, this book does not cover any of these even though the lion's share of personal development time is spent enhancing these skills.

Mental skills are cognitive (IQ) related. This is often how fast you can draw the correct conclusions. These are the data points of every experience (patient and co-worker) that are used to make decisions on what course of action to take. While reading a chart, for example, your cognitive functions notice that a certain test result is off. Your brain then makes a decision to explore that anomaly. Once that decision is made, then the medical skill of recalling past experience and training take over and a course of action takes place. Mental strength is having the experience to know the best decision to make based on several data points. Mental strength is not emotional strength. You may have the ability to process the above anomaly in the manner described and the medical training to prescribe the right course of action, but if just before you made that decision, you recall the last patient with a similar anomaly where you made an incorrect decision in a similar situation, then the emotional trauma of the previous experience will compromise both your mental strength and your medical skills as discussed earlier in the decision-making sequence. What leads to compromising this decision-making is the EQ part that every Clinician has to negotiate through.

Moving forward, this book will be specific in drawing attention to these three areas of skills so as to properly delineate and learn from.

Let's take two Clinicians, Jill and Pam, of the same vocation working on the same floor. Both went to a half-day continuing medical education seminar to keep their certifications. Both of them reported to their peers, tweeted, and posted on Facebook to their friends that they completed their class. When their manager debriefed with both Jill and Pam, she learned that the identical seminar was experienced very differently. Pam was very focused, did each activity specifically as directed by the instructor. Pam shared several observations based on this data with her manager to discuss potential changes they may want to make. The ***purpose*** of the training was met. Jill, however, was distracted. She had a personal situation with her boyfriend that was not going well and her mind kept wandering towards solutions for the relationship. While she completed all of the activities like Pam, her focus was on and off, and as a result, she was inconsistent in what she actually learned. As expected, her follow up session with the manager was not very productive. It was hard for her manager to know whether any of the issues Jill had were related to the seminar or her lack of focus. Jill's experience, though commendable for the four-hours she took off her busy day, was not nearly as good of a learning experience as that of Pam. Although both Clinicians put in four hours of training, clearly the value to each was totally different.

This chapter is included in this book because EQ comes into play in your ability to learn as well, not just to perform during a shift. Healthcare is a unique vocation in that there are dozens of medical and mental skills required, often taking a 'team' to effectively treat a patient. There is a lot to learn and each patient experience has the full capacity to be a *seminar,* like the ones Jill and Pam attended. **Yet, Clinicians often are not trained or incentivized to process patient experiences as learning seminars individually or collectively so that collective experience is enhanced such that future patients can benefit from**. There is a lot to learn in this multidiscipline vocation of healthcare.

"I learned that courage was not the absence of fear, but the triumph over it. The brave man is not he who does not feel afraid, but he who conquers that fear." -Nelson Mandela

In this chapter, we explore the art and science of learning. The objective is to have you become very comfortable with processing experiences on the floor as learning experiences, especially stressful times, and then to be able to have a framework to process any mistakes into learning that can stick with you for future patients. Constant learning needs to be fully engrained as a way of protocol for every Clinician. The richness in daily patient experiences will never come close to what you may learn in a seminar, offsite in a classroom. This paradigm shift is one that must be made. When an airplane crashes, multiple stakeholders, the NTSB, airline, parts-makers, police, all collaborate to preserve the site and extract as much as possible the cause of the crash mostly so that the learning can be very quickly transferred to practice to prevent a future crash. Healthcare needs to adopt a similar approach, not just when something goes wrong, but all the time. Learning is an emotional exercise as much as it is a technical exercise. It takes courage to ask yourself, "What could I/we have done better?" We have addressed the EQ component of being a Clinician, but wanted to focus on the technical components of good learning in this chapter. Healthcare, after all, is a multi-disciplinary field of constant changes, and mistakes do happen.

Learning can occur proactively, as demonstrated by Pam in the example above. This can be done using a trial and error approach to figure out what works and what does not. Learning can also be reactive, where a challenging situation occurs as a by-product of the experience, often unplanned, but equally valuable for learning. As there is so much to learn in healthcare, it is critical that to be good at caregiving, you must inherently be good at learning.

Myth about Learning

There is a misperception about learning that has spread quite rapidly. It is from Malcolm Gladwell's 10,000 Rule from his book *Outliers: The Story of Success*, which, incidentally, is a great read. Many coaches in all sports are convincing athletes that based on the research of the book, in which Gladwell has suggested that it takes 10,000 hours to fully learn a skill and become an expert at it, that volume (repetition) exclusively is the key to mastery. This has resulted in the false premise of assuming that simply putting in the hours gets you the learning and experience needed to master your craft. It can lead to complacency in the kind of proactive and systemized learning we are suggesting healthcare needs. In the example of the seminar for Jill and Pam, clearly those four hours were not equal. Similarly, it could be argued that it may take Jill several four-hour sessions to accomplish what Pam did in her one session.

What Gladwell actually said was that it takes 10,000 hours to be a phenom, of which there are literally only a handful in the world; men and women who consistently perform at extra-ordinary levels and are often known by one name like Jordan, Elway, Mozart, Phelps, and Tiger.

While we fully appreciate the need for training, the point worth reiterating here is that you must make a distinction in your learning between 'logging in the hours' and 'proactive systemized learning constantly.' Focused learning on the job is priceless with the reward being better care for future patients. We show you how to do the latter in this chapter, which will allow you to be a much smarter learner and Clinician, optimizing the limited time you have.

"You must do the thing you think you cannot do." -Eleanor Roosevelt

Traditional Learning

Most of us have formally learned in the same general methodology. It was the methodology used in most schools at all levels across the world. In the broadest sense, the methodology is based on academic models of memory and testing. Information was given to you in a classroom or other setting, and then you demonstrated that you acquired that knowledge at that specific time period (for example, a semester) by being tested on examinations by answering questions. We concede we are over simplifying academia, but only to underscore the point that we believe learning has historically been very flawed. How you were taught is how we think we need to learn. This is a false assumption. We have convinced ourselves that vocational learning occurs in some formal place with someone *teaching* it to us. We were rarely taught to process our experiences, especially challenging ones, as a rich source of knowledge to build on and grow.

As an adult, you learn best at the *point of need*. This means that if you are going to build a cabinet in your house this upcoming weekend, then the best time in your life to learn about building cabinets are the next few days just before the weekend. Could you have learned a few weeks ago? Yes. Could you learn a few weeks from today? Yes. But now is the best time to learn because you have a need this weekend that necessitates knowledge. Your emotions and appetite to learn are at a peak. In the traditional learning model that most of us have been taught, the need is a false need – it's an examination at a specified time in the academic pipeline – not a true application of what you have learned in the semester. Some estimate that people forget almost all the courses they took in college within five years of graduating, often because what they have learned in the five years after graduating was much more experiential and relevantly applicable to needs (job). For Clinicians, the opportunity to learn in every clinical experience is not just a philosophical argument, but very much a real one.

Another reason we believe why traditional learning models are flawed is that they typically have been designed to fit only one style of personality and learning. Extensive research in adult learning over the past 20 years has revealed that there are, in fact, many styles of learning, with no one being 'better' than the other. The key is to find out what type of learner you are and then seek to process your learning in that modality. Given this, it is important for healthcare providers to find learning models that are flexible enough to match their style.

Some good questions worth asking yourself are: how good of a learner are you? What methodology do you follow to learn? How often does learning translate to desired better outcomes?

Learning Styles

According to Neil Fleming's VARK Model, there are several learning styles. It is important to know your style. Note that your style may vary based on the specific need you have, the urgency of that need, and the availability of resources to learn. The styles are:

- Visual (spatial): You prefer using pictures, images, and spatial understanding.
- Aural (auditory-musical): You prefer using sound and music.
- Verbal (linguistic): You prefer using words, both in speech and writing.
- Physical (kinesthetic): You prefer using your body, hands and sense of touch.
- Logical (mathematical): You prefer using logic, reasoning and systems.
- Social (interpersonal): You prefer to learn in groups or with other people.
- Solitary (intrapersonal): You prefer to work alone and use self-study.

What is your style and how can you modify how you learn to match this style? This could be either on your own or with a coach.

Learning Agility

What is actually more important than knowing your learning style is to have the desire to want to learn all the time. This is called having *learning agility*. Athletes who perform optimally have very high learning agility. In general, people who have high learning agility live healthier and more successful lives. They view almost all experiences as an opportunity to learn and, in fact, embrace weaknesses or mistakes as *the* reason to work harder and more effectively.

In sports, we have seen incredible transformations in athletes who previously thought they were the hardest working athletes in their sport only to realize that they had not been learning nearly as effectively as they could have been. **Repetition is not experience, constant learning is**. As a Clinician, unlike an athlete, you have much more to gain as do your patients. So, make a commitment to learn from every experience and learn to apply that learning to the next experience. Let us show you how.

"I've missed more than 9000 shots in my career. I've lost almost 300 games. 26 times, I've been trusted to take the game winning shot and missed. I've failed over and over and over again in my life. And that is why I succeed." -Michael Jordan

Learning Methodology

There is both an art and a science to learning. In the methodology we recommend, there is a blend between the art and science as well as a key third dimension designed to make sure that once you have learned something, there is a process to then make it stick. We call this last step the 7-7 Rule.

Given that so much of learning in healthcare is haphazard (never knowing which patient will present the challenge), when something 'clicks' it is even more important to find ways to make that something last for as long as possible.

The Art of Learning

The art is the emotional component that we have already discussed in Chapter 2. In both proactive and reactive learning, it is important to be in GREEN in order to learn. If you are YELLOW (as was likely the case with Jill) or RED (as was the case with the examples in Chapter 1), then your learning is compromised before your patient experience even begins. The first step for Jill could have been to take her emotional temperature on her way to the seminar and upon realizing she was YELLOW, to then read her YELLOW card to allow her to get back to GREEN before entering the room. In addition, Jill may be well served to also have YELLOW CARD-LIKE focal memories during her seminar with brief and intermittent breaks to review her YELLOW CARD. This is much better than just going through the motions of being present and going through the motions that Jill ended up doing.

"You're going to make mistakes. The key is to learn from them as fast as possible and make changes as soon as you can. That's not always easy to do because ego and pride get in the way." -Tiger Woods

The Science of Learning

Once in GREEN, then the science of learning comes into play for both proactive learning (planned experiences) and reactive learning (unplanned experiences).

Below is a very simple 5-Step general template that we encourage you to use dozens of times, or for at least six months. This template has instructions for completion. There is a 'clean version' of the template at the end of this chapter for you to complete and a completed template example provided as well.

Exercise: Learning Template Instructions

1. **Problem Statement:** Each learning can only have ONE problem. You cannot have two or more problems in one template. A common barrier to learning is the tangled-up nature of how we think about a problem. In addition, the problem statement is brief and NO SOLUTION OR CAUSE can be part of this statement.

2. **Symptoms of Problem:** There should not be more than 3 symptoms and if there are actually more, then pick the top 3. In addition, each symptom should be described in less than 5 words.

3. **Potential Root Causes:** Each root cause must be directly related to the symptom. If it is not, then it is not a root cause. There should not be more than 3 potential root causes and if there are actually more, then pick the top 3. In addition, each root cause should be described in less than 5 words.

4. **Sources for Solution:** There should not be more than 3 sources and if there are actually more, then pick the top 3. In addition, each source should be described in less than 5 words.

5. **Potential Solutions:** Each solution must directly address the root cause in step 3. The only way to know this is to try the solution and see if an impact is made to the symptoms in Step 2. There should not be more than 3 solutions and if there are more, then pick the top 3. In addition, each solution should be described in less than 5 words. These solutions could be from one or more of the sources in Step 4.

Exercise: Learning Template

1. **Problem Statement:** _____

2. **Symptoms of Problem:**

   a. _____

   b. _____

   c. _____

3. **Potential Root Causes:**

   a. _____

   b. _____

   c. _____

4. **Sources for Solution:**

   a. _____

   b. _____

   c. _____

5. **Potential Solutions:**

   a. _____

   b. _____

   c. _____

Sample Completed Learning Template (Pam)

1. **Problem Statement:** <u>As my day goes on I find it harder to remember the finer details of a new patient's history.</u>

2. **Symptoms of Problem:**

   a. <u>Having to go back and clarify details with the patient</u>

   b. <u>Documentation suffers</u>

   c.

3. **Potential Root Causes:**

   a. <u>Distracted by cumulative pressure</u>

   b. <u>Still thinking about tasks or problems with my last patient</u>

   c. <u>Thinking about what I need to do next</u>

4. **Sources for Solution:**

   a. <u>Talk with my colleagues/director</u>

   b. <u>Examine how I do things at the beginning of the day</u>

   c.

5. **Potential Solutions:**

   a. <u>Using micro focus while talking with my patients to be more present and hear more</u>

   b. <u>Writing brief notes to jog my memory</u>

   c. <u>Taking my emotional temperature and taking corrective steps before going into a new patient's room.</u>

Healthcare presents some of the best opportunities to be learners because each patient really is a puzzle to solve, a 'problem' to dissect. The *best* time to learn is right after a challenging patient experience. Just like building the deck on the weekend, yes, you can learn about a challenging patient experience a few weeks from now, but very shortly after the experience is the best time to learn. Usually, the best time to learn is within 24 hours of a challenging experience. After this, research shows that the emotional state (art) has altered significantly and you have moved on to other parts of your priorities or life in general. With so much stimuli in today's world and on the work floor, your best appetite to learn, i.e., learning agility, is at its peak immediately after as you wrestle with the *why* of some of the decisions you made. Using the template, the first four steps could be done immediately. This is what makes a good learner. However, our general tendency is to skip the first four steps and immediately get to the solutions. A hasty approach often results in poor learning, creation of additional issues, and most notably, reinforcement of all bad habits (remember what the brain does with bad memories from Chapter 2).

From an emotional perspective, the other great and not to be overlooked power of immediate learning is that once the 'framework' of learning is initiated, the trauma dilutes itself. If there is no learning from a challenging experience, our brain stores that experience in the 'negative' memory bank, allowing it to mutate into future anxiety.

"Success does not consist in never making mistakes, but in never making the same one a second time." -George Bernard Shaw

There is a reason almost all professional athletes have a coach. There is recognition of the dozens of moving body parts in most sports and that all of them have to come together for a good performance. Another set of eyes from a trained coach is primarily a training aid for athletes to do exactly what we are talking about above – to see what is wrong, figure out what is causing it, explore options, and get it corrected. Coaches use videos and all kinds of technology to analyze every situation with the goal of making them better for the next performance. Clinicians do not have the luxury of a coach, but can certainly make themselves better learners.

The 7-7 Rule

The 7-7 Rule states that in order to instill new learning, it has to be experienced in 7 different ways at 7 different times within 7 days. The 7-7 Rule is designed to help you make sure that new learning has the optimal stickiness factor, so that it can be imprinted and retrieved by your brain when it is needed the most. It is designed to prevent you from going to work without leveraging key learnings from yesterday or the recent past by forgetting what you learned at the very moment you needed to remember it. Done correctly, it can significantly cut down those 10,000 hours of mastery required. Repetition is an archaic way of imprinting new skills. In the world we live in today, the sheer volume of experiences vying for mind-share is enormous. A Clinician has to give performance learning an added and proactive nudge to make sure it gets imprinted. *Note that one of the 7 ways has to be a negative imprint.* That is, it has to be the incorrect way of doing things, or simply put, your old way of doing things. The 7-7 Rule is based on three concepts that are being weaved together for the first time in this book.

1. Structure and Accountability

The first of the three is research done by Dr. Gail Matthews on accomplishing goals. Take a look at the table below.

Table 1. Achieving Goal Success

	Group 1	Group 2-3	Group 4	Group 5
Think about goals	✓	✓	✓	✓
Write about goals	✗	✓	✓	✓
Share with a friend	✗	✗	✓	✓
Weekly **progress report** to friend	✗	✗	✗	✓
Success Rate	**43%**	**56%**	**64%**	**76%**

Her study demonstrates powerfully the value of having structure and peer support in accomplishing desired goals. The more of both, the better the chances of achieving goals. The same applies to making something new stick. In healthcare, it may be as simple as having a wall-board where each person writes down what he/she learned before leaving his/her shift. Or telling a peer about your learning and asking him/her to remind you of it for a period of time in a learning-buddy system.

2. Kinesiology

The second concept is based on the neuroscience of kinesiology, the study of human kinetics combined with memory formation, specifically of new neuropathways (ways of thinking). It essentially suggests that while learning, and in order to create stronger imprints (new neuropathways) in our brain, all five senses (hear, feel, sight, smell, taste) must be collectively involved in the learning. In other words, the more engaged and experiential your learning, the greater the probability of it sticking.

3. 3-1 EQ Visualization Ratio

The third concept is based on the 3-1 EQ Visualization Ratio. This suggests that three EQ-based repetitions (non-physical) are equivalent to one physical repetition of an exercise. For example, if you are laying in bed, and you combine powerful visualization with imagination to recall a new learning three times, it is as good to your brain as actually doing the exercise physically once. In fact, researchers at the Cleveland Clinic Foundation demonstrated that mental training alone can sometimes induce muscle strength and new patterns.

It is often implied when using the term visualization that you are referring to the future. You are often told to visualize success, or a goal, or a desired outcome, before it has happened. There are so many good quotes out there from inspiring people on the power of dreaming about something better in the future. This is all good. It is healthy to lay in bed dreaming about something you have not done, something you want to achieve, or something no one has thought of. The emotional power from these kinds of exercises is tremendous, often resulting in confidence, courage, and hope, which are priceless emotions to have during your work day.

Because the past is filled with both positive and negative experiences, unlike the future where neither has occurred, we tend to not visualize or dream about the past. It seems counter intuitive at first pass. Why waste time visualizing something you have already done? *Well, we argue that visualizing something successful that you have already done is actually more empowering than visualizing something in the future where you have not done it yet. It is easier to visualize the past simply because you were there, you have all the details of the experience when you had an "aha" moment or events where you performed at your best.* You know where you were, how it happened, who else was there, and how it felt like emotionally. The past seems to get a bad rap as a place where only bad experiences exist and as such, we forget what a great place it can be to give us confidence, courage, and hope – as described in crafting the YELLOW and RED cards. Instead of standing in front of the door to a patient visualizing a positive experience you want to have (that does not yet exist), why not visualize a similar recent experience that went great from your YELLOW card? The 3:1 EQ Ratio is, therefore, a powerful tool that Clinicians should learn as an integral part of that constant learning and strive to perform at high levels in front of all patients. During a shift, however, it is hard to visualize anything as so much is going on. This is why the information on your GREEN, YELLOW, and RED cards is all about data points from the past since they are so much easier to recall, than trying to visualize something in the future. **We recommend that in lieu if visualizing the positive experience that you want to have, which has not happened yet, visualize a similar one you have already had and simply trust that you can duplicate.**

Learning or having an 'aha' moment is not the end game. Too often, we find ourselves making the same mistakes and having to learn the same solutions over and over again. Just ask any coach and he or she will tell you that it takes a great deal of reinforcement and thus time, especially with brand new learning, to get them to stick. The root cause of this incomplete learning is that not enough has been done to reinforce the learning at the time it was best to reinforce it.

Applying the 7-7 Rule

The 7-7 Rule states that in order to instill new learning, it has to be experienced in 7 different ways at 7 different times, incorporating all the three research-based concepts of the 7-7 Rule.

Here is an experience after the physician (Bob) was certified in EQ:

> At work in the ED, when the charge nurse says, "Dr. there is a pediatric trauma alert in room 4." I get up and walk to the room. (Pediatric trauma can be a hot button for some docs.) I check my EQ temp before I walk in the room. Calming breath to my abs before game time. I walk in the room and I see a mother in her mid20s holding an infant carrier. On the stretcher is an infant, awake, crying, pink. The mother looks like she could break down. She tells me the history; she had placed the baby in the carrier and when she was walking she got off balance and the baby fell from the carrier. No loss of consciousness. Baby cried immediately. No change in behavior. After assessing the baby and determining that there are no signs of any significant injury, I focused on the other patient in the room. That being the mother. She was highly distressed. She was worried about her baby, she was worried that people would blame her if he was injured, etc. I put my arm around her and said slowly and calmly, "Its ok. It was just an accident. Accidents happen. He doesn't have any injuries from the fall. I want to keep an eye on you both for a little bit

to make sure everything is going to be fine." I checked on them both over the next 30 minutes. The mother calmed down, the baby was easily comforted and stopped crying. Mom felt comfortable that her baby was fine and all went home happy.

Bob had been certified in EQ. He learned all the tools, but the magic does not happen in learning. It happens when learning is applied by imprinting those learnings so they can show up during his *game-time* – the patient experience.

So, Bob had to learn to take his EQ temperature and breathe, skills as a skilled ER physician he had not learned before. He had to consciously practice the ACT model of breathing in 7 different ways at 7 different times (one of them being consciously doing it the old way to remind him to feel what he does not want to feel). He had to do this to make sure that he had less chances of reverting to the 'old way' of just going into the room and relying only on medical skills to navigate the patient experience. As an example, here are Bob's 7-7 action steps to imprint the skills he used:

1. Do ACT breathing first thing after waking up.
2. Set alarm for every 3 hours to practice ACT breathing.
3. Practice taking EQ temperature at same alarm.
4. Take one day and not practice these tools to gauge the difference.
5. Practice consciously the difference between fast breath (stress) and slower breath (calm), and monitor how the body and mind operates in both conditions.
6. Tell at least 2 nurses about what you learned and are doing.
7. While laying in bed, visualize the completed day and the good job you did breathing and taking your EQ temperature.

Bob started doing this immediately after he learned them. You can see Bob has incorporated all three concepts in his 7-7 Rule after learning the ACT model and learning to take his EQ temperature. Note also that many modalities and senses are being used. This method allows for imprinting of new neuropathways to re-direct the proverbial 'old habits' which are nothing more than strongly entrenched neuropathways. The more senses engaged in different modes in the imprinting process, the 7-7 process, then the more re-directing of old ways into new ones. This is a very different way of learning as most athletes and Clinicians focus purely on learning, and either not on imprinting that learning or using *volume* or repetition for that imprinting. The latter is a very poor and inefficient way to imprint your learning, but used by many simply because it *seems* like the right thing to do.

Obviously, though these modalities worked for Bob, they may not work for you. You have to decide what you can do, based on your own past positive learning, to make sure enough diversity is included that is personalized to your own style of learning to make it stick.

In proactive learning, it is much easier to implement both the learning methodology (i.e., the art and science of learning) and the 7-7 Rule, if there actually is a goal/purpose you have with each patient. Having a purpose almost always means having a way to measure your output. It can be diagnosis, treatment, outcome, patient experience, or just how you felt. If you have a PURPOSE for your experience, then you are inherently opening yourself up to learning because if that purpose is not met, then the opportunity to apply the learning methodology and 7-7 rule also exists.

Athletes who perform well (being in a zone) talk of how slow everything goes, and conversely, those who do not, talk about how fast everything is. Time is neither faster nor slower – your thinking, dictated by your emotions, is. The cost of not learning can be very high. If you can set a purpose and learn constantly, then you are preventing the prefrontal lobes from sounding a compromising alarm in your brain which dilutes your ability to make the right decision.

"Life isn't about finding yourself. Life is about creating yourself." -George Bernard Shaw

Learning to Evaluate

We also recommend that every challenging experience ends with using the Goal Post Model. This model helps you visually keep track of each experience with respect to each of the three skills mentioned earlier in the chapter. Consider this your own personal performance review.

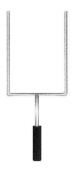

Figure 9. The Goal Post

The Goal Post Model is quite simple. As you can see in the picture, the goal post looks like a football goal post. After the challenging experience, simply draw the goal post in your note book. Write down on the bottom left side of the post, just 1-3 things that went well in the experience. On the bottom right side of the post, write 1-3 things that did not. Then on top of the goal post, notice three areas of space: inside the goal post, to the left of it, and to the right of it.

Inside the goal post, in the middle, write down only 1-3 things from a medical skill perspective that you need to work on. On the left, write down only 1-3 things from a mental skill perspective that you need to work on. On the right, write down only 1-3 things from an EQ skill perspective that you need to work on – things like how often you felt YELLOW or RED, whether you were present (next chapter) or how quickly or poorly you were able to get back to GREEN.

Do this immediately after your experience and consider the day incomplete if this is not done. Review it just before your next day or with others. Use the learning template on the areas that you feel you underperformed and get to the real root causes and subsequent solutions. It is that simple. Professional athletes, who have very short careers, live by some version of this model after each game. You are doing something infinitely more important in healthcare.

In basketball, there is a sheet of paper that is printed and given to the coach at the end of each quarter that lists all the players who played, how many minutes they played, points scored, rebounds had, assists made, etc. This is used by the coaches to make adjustments and manage the game. Similarly, in healthcare, you need to also assess your performance and do the same thing in order to grow.

Complete Your Learning Template

Exercise: Learning Template

1. **Problem Statement:** _____

2. **Symptoms of Problem:**
   a. _____
   b. _____
   c. _____

3. **Potential Root Causes:**
   a. _____
   b. _____
   c. _____

4. **Sources for Solution:**
   a. _____
   b. _____
   c. _____

5. **Potential Solutions:**
   a. _____
   b. _____
   c. _____

Exercise: Apply 7-7 Rule

As practice, apply the 7-7 rule to your solutions above:

1. _____
2. _____
3. _____
4. _____
5. _____
6. _____
7. _____

Top 3 Ideas		
I learned from this chapter		
1.		
2.		
3.		
3 Action Steps		
I will take immediately to incorporate the above learning into my day		
1.		
2.		
3.		

Chapter Summary

1. Being a proactive learner can significantly improve the quality of your performance as it will allow you to take charge of your growth with medical, mental, and emotional skills.
2. Learning takes place best when there is a purpose, and there is both an art and a science to it.
3. No work day should be complete without an evaluation of how you performed with medical skills, mental skills, and emotional skills.
4. Everyone has a different learning style and should utilize that style to take advantage of opportunities.
5. Learning is only half of the equation to improvement. The other half is to make that learning stick by incorporating the 7-7 Rule.

Chapter 5

There has never been a shortage of ways to describe happiness. If we are lucky enough to have our basic needs (Maslow) of food, water, shelter and security met, then the pursuit of happiness comes into play. Scientific studies and evidence correlating happy workers to productive workers and high degrees of innovation are abundant and at least 40 years old. There is indisputable evidence suggesting that happy workers or athletes outperform those who are not. Defining happiness to begin with is key to understanding and we can now do it with neuroscience. We now know that Happiness has more to do with the impact of our negative experiences and less to do with happy experiences. Managing negativity (past or present) has more to do with our overall happiness, and less with all the happy moments (past or present) we have had. Happiness is tied to our interpretation of current experiences and that interpretation is personally biased by our past negative experiences.

-Dr. Izzy Justice

Happiness and Focus

You have been introduced to several concepts so far, most notably, that of how your brain makes decisions, EQ, and learning. You now have several tools to incorporate into your work day and personal life. In the next four chapters, we spend time on a few common Clinician scenarios and apply all these concepts, where it matters the most. But before we go there, in this chapter, we discuss two other key concepts of high performance not just in healthcare, but also in life: happiness and focus. A shift at work lasts just a few hours, but your life itself consumes countless hours of both actual time and emotional energy that unequivocally come into play during your shift. Practicing EQ during outside work life creates new neuropathways that during your shift, when you need them most, will not be new.

In the last chapter, you learned about how to learn to avoid those *garbage* hours at work or in training, where you are simply going through the motions repetitively and nothing is being learned, or worse, nothing is being imprinted. You may be doing it just to say you logged in the hours. These *garbage* hours can be further reduced significantly by incorporating EQ in life itself, totally outside of work.

Happiness

This is quite possibly the least considered variable in all of human performance, not just in healthcare, but also in athletic performance. Some of you are no doubt skeptical here. You may ask, "What in the world does personal happiness have to do with my ability to draw blood?" and it is a fair question. It is infinitely more important, however, that you understand what happiness actually is, from a neuroscience perspective.

Some psychologists and philosophers argue that happiness is in fact, the ultimate pursuit. If you are a Clinician, you do it to make yourself happy. If you work at an office, you do it to make money to do something to make you happy. If you play with your child, you do it to make you happy. If you listen to a song or read a book or watch a movie, at its core, you do it all because 'something' inside you makes you feel better. The clothes you chose to wear today, the way you do your hair, what you say – all of it – is an expression of your identity that you hope will either make you directly happy or accepted by others which itself would make you happy. These are activities that chase the dopamine hormone.

Another way to look at this ultimate pursuit is the converse. Who among you pursues activities that make you unhappy? It could even be argued that we intentionally avoid experiences that we know will make us unhappy. So clearly there is a ying-yang effect here of things that we do, or happen to us, that either make us happy or unhappy. Some of these things we choose, but many others we do not choose. You can choose to hug your child, which makes you happy, but you cannot choose when someone screams at you, which makes you unhappy.

There are countless stories of great athletes who suddenly look like they are clueless while performing, only to later find out that they had just lost a loved one a day earlier or a similar personal tragedy. In life, it is not hard to see a decline in work performance when a negative life event, like a divorce or break-up, occurs. On the other hand, it is also noted that people suddenly perform great when 'their personal life' gets in order. In either case, and so many in between the spectrum of something good or bad experiences of life, the Clinicians weight, height, IQ, or medical knowledge does not change considerably, yet can all be impacted by those experiences.

Exercise: Negative Experience

List a time in your life when a negative experience impacted you negatively.

_____

_____

_____

Exercise: Positive Experience

List a time in your life when a positive experience impacted you positively.

_____

_____

_____

You are encouraged to complete the exercises above before proceeding so that what is next can be personal to you.

It is critical for those who seek higher performance to understand the role of happiness in their lives and performance.

The Neuroscience of Happiness

The human body is over 90% fluid. We are essentially a chemical factory with many hormones in our body released from several glands that determine what the composition of 'you' is at any given time. The chemical composition of the mix of hormones is constantly changing, mostly without your control or knowledge. You only find out after the fact by noticing the impact of the new chemical state in, perhaps, how you behaved.

Without giving you all a dissertation, let us simplify it down to two dominant families of hormones: Dopamine and Cortisol. Dopamine is your happy family of hormones and Cortisol is your unhappy family of hormones.

A good question to ask is why, if the ultimate pursuit is happiness, does the cortisol family even exist? Think back to the car coming at you in Chapter 2. In addition, the pursuit of happiness is a very new phenomenon in our evolution as human beings. We were built, as all living creatures are, to primarily defend ourselves and live to survive another day. We were designed so that if we saw a fire on our right, we would immediately, as described in Chapter 2 with the car, turn to our left and run. The same applies to seeing a lion coming at us to eat us, and running the opposite way or figuring out a way to fight it. Until the last 100 years or so, most human beings never traveled more than 50 miles from their place of birth nor lived beyond the age of 40. Our inherent design is not conducive to consistent high performance as that usually means we have to deal with failures constantly. This all happens because of the cortisol family of hormones and, for the most part, we still very much need them to continue to survive.

When the cortisol levels are higher than the dopamine levels, then, generally speaking, we are unhappy. The neurological state of unhappiness is simply that – a higher presence of cortisol than dopamine – which leads the initial neuropathways, and potentially subsequent ones also, to our negative memories so we can decipher the negative stimulus and give it the personal threat rating. New research is showing that four out of five Americans are permanently in this YELLOW state because of negative experiences in the past, recent past, or currently being experienced. It could have been a traumatic childhood experience, or something that happened with a patient last week, or a current health issue with you or a loved one. These experiences release cortisol in your body which creates the stress levels that we call unhappiness. And as already discussed, when in YELLOW or RED state, you can neither physically nor cognitively recollect the medical skills to perform optimally.

"The greatest discovery of all time is that a person can change his future by merely changing his attitude." -Oprah Winfrey

Given that healthcare is already a stressful job (negative experiences releasing cortisol), the brain is constantly compromised to make the best decision you are capable of. And this does not even take into account all that has happened to you in life before you started your shift, all of which is stored in the same brain that you will need in front of your next patient. The idea that happiness can counteract these negative experiences was first explored in performance in the 1920s in the Hawthorne Experiments — something worth googling.

The **Hawthorne studies**, which were conducted by Elton Mayo and Fritz Roethlisberger in the 1920s with workers at the **Hawthorne** plant of the Western Electric Company, were part of an emphasis on socio-psychological aspects of human behavior in organizations. They found that by simply making lights brighter, factory workers 'felt happy' and productivity increased. They played music and the same positive impact on performance resulted.

Since then, neuroscience has emerged to take observations by psychologists; and now be able to explain them using digital imaging of the brain during states of happiness and unhappiness. An incredible amount of new research over the past decade has provided priceless knowledge on how to be happy.

Matt Killingsworth, a Harvard researcher, unveiled a great study on the correlation of happiness to being present. **He essentially showed that most human beings have their mind wondering 60% of the time**. In other words, 60% of the time, your mind is somewhere other than where you physically are, thinking about something else rather than what you are actually doing.

For Clinicians, this is a very troubling statistic and explains "hindsight" – where after the fact you think of doing something better than you did it the first time. In the hindsight, you are more 'present' than the original moment. It cannot possibly be a medical skill issue or mental issue because if it were, you would not be able to think of the better way of doing it after the fact. You already had the skill to do better, but it was compromised by being in YELLOW or RED.

It is part of life's vernacular to hear 'stay in the present' or 'stay in the moment,' but rarely has this been decoded with neuroscience, and even rarer, is how to do it beyond just telling someone to do it.

"Concentration is a fine antidote to anxiety." -Jack Nicklaus

How to be Mindful – Stay in the Moment

For the next section, you will need to be very disciplined and follow the instructions very carefully, exactly as prescribed otherwise you will compromise your own learning. You will need a picture of anything – a person or a place – and something you can eat like a fruit or power bar of some kind.

Being mindful or being in the present means that your neuropathways (thinking) are all correct in accessing the right memories and skills for the moment required.

We know that our thinking is a consequence of our emotions (Chapter 2) which, in turn, is a reaction to stimuli. So, all the changes to that chemical composition of that 90% chemical factory, called the human body, begin with stimuli. Earlier, we learned to trick (self- stimulate) the brain with past positive experiences with the YELLOW and GREEN cards. In the present moment, however, a different way can be used and it is complementary to the cards.

Stimuli enter our cognitive space in only five ways – sight, sound, smell, taste, and feel. All stimuli must go through these channels to have meaning of any kind. To be present, to be in the moment, to be mindful, therefore, is having strong skills with these five sensory channels. It sounds bizarre at first to suggest that you are going to learn to see, hear, taste, smell, or feel – we have been doing this since we were born. But how many of you have actually been taught to enhance these skills?

We know people who are blind who have unbelievable hearing skills, but no biological reason for that enhanced hearing skill. They have simply trained themselves to be better at hearing as a necessity. We may also know people who are deaf, but have incredible sense of feel and sight, yet no biological reason for that other than training themselves to be better at them. The point here is that having a better skill over your entry senses is very much possible and you have simply not explored it because you have not had the need to or do not know how to do it. You will learn now.

Sight

Let us start with the most powerful of the five senses: sight. Take the picture you were asked to have and look at it.

Write down three unique attributes of what you see in that picture:

1. _____
2. _____
3. _____

Look at the picture again now, and write down three additional attributes of what you see in that picture:

4. _____
5. _____
6. _____

Look at the picture again now, and write down three additional attributes of what you see in that picture:

7. _____
8. _____
9. _____

Look at the picture again now, and write down three additional attributes of what you see in that picture:

10. _____
11. _____
12. _____

Look at the picture again now, and write down three additional attributes of what you see in that picture:

13. _____
14. _____
15. _____

If you completed each set of the above exercise, you are probably surprised as you thought you could not come up with new unique attributes.

"You can see a lot by just looking." -Yogi Berra

If you went further, you could probably come up with another 15 attributes. One of the best ways to practice this is to look at the live face of a loved one – a spouse or child – and come up with 50 unique attributes of his or her face only. It is an advanced skill, but can easily be done with any face. You will find yourself noticing every little feature. And in that moment of looking and searching, your mind is in no other place than the present. **This is how you use sight to stay present.** This is how you use sight to focus – which we will discuss at length later in this chapter. Just imagine ALL the things that are available to the eye during your shift on a clinic floor that you simply do not notice. If you can pick out 15 attributes in just one picture, and be present, how many could you pick up on each patient's face, that could equally keep your mind from wandering and be in the present? Using this technique to be present allows your neuropathways not to go to the negative memory bank and redirect it to the memory of your skills to make the right decision.

Sound

The next most powerful of the five senses is sound. For this, just stay wherever you are reading this book and close your eyes before each set and zone in on just listening.

Close your eyes and hear three unique sounds wherever you presently are. Write them down below:

1. _____
2. _____
3. _____

Close your eyes again and hear three additional unique sounds wherever you presently are. Write them down below:

4. _____
5. _____
6. _____

Close your eyes again and hear three additional unique sounds wherever you presently are. Write them down below:

7. _____
8. _____
9. _____

Close your eyes again and hear three additional unique sounds wherever you presently are. Write them down below:

10. _____
11. _____
12. _____

Close your eyes again and hear three additional unique sounds wherever you presently are. Write them down below:

13. _____
14. _____
15. _____

If you completed each set of the above exercise, you are probably surprised as you thought you could not come up with new unique sounds.

"That's been one of my mantras - focus and simplicity. Simple can be harder than complex: You have to work hard to get your thinking clean to make it simple. But it's worth it in the end because once you get there, you can move mountains." -Steve Jobs

If you went further, you could probably hear more sounds. This is an advanced skill, but can easily be done by practicing literally anywhere, at any time. Eventually, you will find yourself noticing every little sound the way perhaps a skilled blind person does. And in that moment of listening and searching for new sounds, your mind is in no other place than the present. **This is how you use sound to stay present.** This is how you use sound to focus, which we will discuss at length later in this chapter. Just imagine ALL the things that are available to hear during your shift that you simply do not choose to hear. If you can pick out 15 sounds just where you are now, and be present, how many could you pick up on in a patient's room, that could equally keep your mind from wandering and be in the present?

Feel

Next is feel. Like sound, just stay wherever you are reading this book and close your eyes before each set and zone in on just feeling something on your body.

Close your eyes and feel three unique sensations all over your body wherever you presently are. Write them down below:

1. _____
2. _____
3. _____

Close your eyes and feel three additional unique sensations all over your body wherever you presently are. Write them down below:

4. _____
5. _____
6. _____

Close your eyes and feel three additional unique sensations all over your body wherever you presently are. Write them down below:

7. _____
8. _____
9. _____

Close your eyes and feel three additional unique sensations all over your body wherever you presently are. Write them down below:

10. _____
11. _____
12. _____

Close your eyes and feel three additional unique sensations all over your body wherever you presently are. Write them down below.

13. _____
14. _____
15. _____

If you completed each set of the above exercise, you are probably surprised as you thought you could not come up with new unique sensations to feel.

If you went further, you could probably come up with another 15 sensations. This is not an advanced skill and can be practiced anywhere, anytime. You will find yourself feeling everything on you, perhaps even the weight of a pen in your hand while walking on the floor. And in that moment of feeling and searching, your mind is in no other place than the present. **This is how you use feel to stay present.** This is how you use feel to focus, which we will discuss at length later in this chapter. Just imagine ALL the things that are available to feel during your shift that you simply do not notice. Perhaps it's the glove you are wearing, or your grip on an instrument in your hand. If you can pick out 15 attributes in just where you are now, and be present, how many could you pick up while being with a patient, that could equally keep your mind from wandering and be in the present?

Taste

The next sense is taste. For this, you will need that power bar mentioned earlier. Just stay wherever you are reading this book and close your eyes before each set and zone in on just tasting.

Close your eyes and take a small bite of whatever you have and eat it the way you would normally eat and notice three unique tastes of what you ate. Write them down below:

1. _____
2. _____
3. _____

Close your eyes again, take another bite and notice three additional unique tastes. Write them down below:

4. _____
5. _____
6. _____

Close your eyes again, take another bite and notice three additional unique tastes. Write them down below:

7. _____
8. _____
9. _____

If you completed each set of the above exercise, you are probably surprised as you thought you could not come up with new unique tastes.

If you went further, you could probably come up with several more tastes in flavor or texture or the way it sits in your mouth. This is an advanced skill, but can easily be done by practicing literally anywhere, at any time, and especially when you eat – which for most of us is at least three times a day. Why not practice this every single time you eat? Eventually, you will find yourself noticing every little taste, the way perhaps a skilled person like a sommelier does. And in that moment of tasting and searching for new tastes, your mind is in no other place than the present. **This is how you use taste to stay present.** This is how you use taste to focus, which we discuss at length later in this chapter. Just imagine ALL the things that are available (from what you drink and eat) to taste during each day, that you simply do not choose to really taste. Why waste that experience since you have to do it anyway? If you can pick out six tastes just with one type of food, and be present, how many could you pick up on each sip or bite if you tasted what you drank or ate, that could equally keep your mind from wandering and be in the present?

Smell

This is difficult to do in book format, and in a room or house. It is best to practice this when outside at a restaurant or outdoor event. Do the same thing as for the previous four senses: close your eyes and seek out three new smells at a time till you get to 12. On a clinic floor, if you engage your sense of smell, you can actually pick up many smells. Perhaps that of medicine, equipment, of patients, etc. And again, by engaging in this sense, you are focusing your mind to respond to the present moment, not wander, and give you a path to lower cortisol by allowing dopamine levels to increase.

What is critical to understand is that being in the moment is a function of your senses. Engaging your sensory organs in this manner allows you to not wander, which, according to Killingsworth's research, is the most powerful way to be happy in any given moment. **The happiness comes from the change in neuropathways from a subconscious one where a negative stimulus searches negative memories, to being present**

where the focus of being present redirects the neuropathway from an instinctive negative path to critical thinking and necessary skills to make the best decision. It is a temporary stop-gap measure that, at least for that *game-time* experience when you need to be at your best, you are allowing yourself the best chance to make the best decision.

This is the same physiological mechanism in play when you are on vacation. Often times, you will go to a place like the beach or mountains. You find that relaxing. The reason is that your senses, all of them, are experiencing a heightened engagement because of the uniqueness of the stimuli of the environment. In other words, the exercises that were just done above with the five senses are happening naturally. Your eyes are looking at the beach, hearing the sounds of the waves, feeling the salty breeze that is common in ocean air. All these sensations cause you to be present, thinking of what you are experiencing instead of what happened the week before or what needs to happen when you return.

The same is said of artists who go to exotic places to search for inspiration. They might go to a cabin in the mountains, for example. The view of trees, greenery, air, natural sounds, all do the same thing for the artists. They keep them present and happy, allowing them to write the lyrics to the song, or paint, or write a book.

What is important to understand is that the inspiration or happiness is happening because senses are engaged fully, and going to a far-away location is a good way of doing it, but by no means the only way. It is possible to be that mindful and inspired wherever you are if you can learn to engage with your senses.

It is impossible, and not necessary, to be a perfectly happy person to perform at a high level; but it is necessary to be able to use your senses to be exactly where you need to be while doing your job so that your negative life experiences do not compromise your ability to make the best decision you are capable of, and not in hindsight. Using such techniques as being mindful (being present while with a patient) is the most effective way to suspend some of life challenges and concurrently manage your neuropathways and chemical composition to allow you to bring out the best you've got.

"Every great player has learned the two C's: how to concentrate and how to maintain composure." -Byron Nelson

FOCUS

Being mindful in the manner described allows you to be focused at the task at hand, and not on the past or future, but in the present moment. Focus is the term often used to describe an athlete who is playing in a zone, executing every move physically, mentally, and emotionally to the best ability.

Once present, there are additional ways to complement the senses that are more mental in order to be even further focused. Being mindful can allow these focal thoughts to be very powerful tools to use during your day.

1. SKILL FOCAL THOUGHT

Once you are in the moment, then it is time to work on building your focus skills and becoming a better Clinician.

A focal thought is one specific medical or mental skill you can use in your day. Depending on where your clinical practice falls on the spectrum, your skill thought may be more of a technical skill or perhaps more of a cognitive awareness. For example, the skill thought used while putting in a chest tube will be different from that used while teasing out the details of a child's seizure history.

Whatever the skill focal point is, it must be very directly related to that patient or clinical scenario. It usually is a thought that helps you remember something that you are just learning, or a best practice you are wanting to adopt.

Exercise: Skill Focal Thoughts

Write down some specific Skill Focal Thoughts (SFT) for next week:

Focal Thought for Patients: _____

Focal Thought for Co-workers: _____

Focal Thought for Family: _____

"All that we are is the result of what we have thought." -Buddha

2. EQ FOCAL THOUGHT

Similar to the skill focal thought, an EQ focal thought is much simpler. It is an EMOTIONAL focal thought. It usually is just one word or a very short phrase for that day or week, like a mantra. Its purpose is to get you to relax and even enjoy your day. It may be the name of your collegiate mascot, your favorite past experience, your favorite song, your spouse or children, your favorite color, or anything that works for you. The purpose of your EQ Focal thought is to have an operating mantra for the entire day no matter what happens. Your ability to revisit this mantra is a measure of your mindfulness and emotional strength. Catch yourself forgetting it. Change it up for each day. Professional athletes do this all the time.

Exercise: EQ Focal Thoughts

Make a list of all the EQ Focal Thoughts that come to mind and use them for your next shift:

a. _____

b. _____

c. _____

d. _____

e. _____

f. _____

g. _____

h. _____

i. _____

j. _____

"Doing the best at this moment puts you in the best place for the next moment." -Oprah Winfrey

3. MACRO FOCUS

Macro focus is an emotionally light way to stay present using your senses as described earlier. It may be to notice the trees, clouds, wind, lawns, ponds, flowers, paintings on wall, clothes people wear, and such. Macro focus is the type of focus required as soon as you enter the clinical facility. Once you pass the entrance threshold of the facility, you are now a professional Clinician trusted to make the best decisions for each patient. You are no longer all your other roles in life.

A fundamental premise in focus is that a conscious effort to think about one thing is a subconscious effort to not think about another thing.

If you choose to notice the big oak tree just outside the entrance doors, then you are subconsciously choosing to not think about the work you have just left or have to do afterwards. You can use all your senses to macro focus. It is important to keep this focus light and make sure it is not the type that drains you emotionally or mentally. It can be smelling the food in the cafeteria while you get your coffee, seeing the shape of clouds, feeling the wind on your body, or hearing birds chirp. This is all light and allows you to be present as described earlier. It is to be used **in between** *game-time* experiences (the latter is when you are with a patient and required to make good decisions).

During the day, macro focus should be the exclusive focus between patients, with the only exception being when you have a YELLOW or RED situation where you will need to breathe and rely on your YELLOW or RED cards. This should complement your EQ focal thought and go hand-in-hand to manage the cortisol and dopamine battle going on in your body.

"Knowing is not enough, we must apply. Willing is not enough, we must do." -Bruce Lee

4. MICRO FOCUS

Micro focus is mindfulness (being present) and is different from macro focus in that micro is a much deeper focus, not light at all. It is a laser-type of focus on a very specific task or spot. Because it is heavier, it is only recommended once you are face to face with a patient or a critical experience (*game-time*). An example is to use sight skills to notice the facial features of your patient. It might also be to feel the grip in every part of your hand and fingers on whatever you have in your hand, or to feel your feet in shoes sensing every inch of the ground underneath. It can even be to sense the saliva in your mouth or quality of air going into your mouth and lungs. **When you are in your *game-time*, with a patient, about to process the needs of the patient, that is the time when all the focus has to be on the patient and nothing else**. Not what happened with the last patient, last week, what is happening at home, or whatever else negative is in your life. Thus, it is important to micro focus using the techniques of mindfulness to make you the happiest, and be in the most present of states to do just that.

It is imperative that you not start micro focus until you are really with a patient. Using micro focus between patients will deplete your emotional energy and you will be exhausted before the day is up. Between patients is when to use macro focus, the light mindfulness technique to still be present. You are still on the clock and other important decisions have to be made too.

"Tell me and I forget, teach me and I may remember, involve me and I learn." -Benjamin Franklin

Top 3 Ideas
I learned from this chapter
1.
2.
3.
3 Action Steps
I will take immediately to incorporate the above learning into my day
1.
2.
3.

Chapter Summary

1. Happiness is a chemical state dictated by the battle between the family of hormones of cortisol (fear) and dopamine (happy).

2. Being present or mindful is a neurologically proven technique to be happy in the moment, increasing dopamine over cortisol and allowing your body to mentally recall a skill and make the best decision.

3. The five senses are an under-utilized asset that, when used to be present, can allow for powerful ways to focus.

4. A clinical setting, full of stimuli of sight, sound, feel, smell, and taste is a great place to engage all your senses to be mindful, an advantage over other vocations.

5. There are skill focus thoughts, EQ focal thoughts, macro and micro focus that collectively can form a powerful emotional strength framework to get you to perform at your best.

Chapter 6

"Be the change that you wish to see in the world." -Mahatma Gandhi

Old Way vs. New Way

In the preceding chapters, we shared the key tools to help you increase your EQ and perform at your best each day. It is time to shift from these concepts to the application of them to you specifically. This entire chapter is a 'journal entry' from Robert Driver, MD. He shares first-hand about how he came to EQ, and his transformation from the 'old way' of doing things to the 'new way' using EQ. In the next chapter, we leverage Robert's candid sharing to build a plan for your *game day* and shift from your 'old way' to your 'new way' with EQ.

"No one cares how much you know, until they know how much you care." -Theodore Roosevelt

When I first met with Dr. Izzy to talk about writing an EQ book for healthcare, I was at the end of my rope. After 17 years in medicine, I was burned out. I had two young kids, had recently lost both of my parents after prolonged illnesses, and was in the middle of a divorce. My entire life was in the midst of change. I decided to pitch the idea of adapting Izzy's program for athletes to healthcare workers and the emergency department to maybe save someone else's future. I felt that mine was already spent. My career in emergency medicine was coming to an end, because I couldn't do it any longer.

"I love the idea. But to write this together, I am going to need you to become EQ certified."

That didn't seem like too much to ask so I agreed. I spent several months reading and studying and learning, and most importantly, applying what I learned. First with my kids, then at work. So, let me tell you about last weekend. I worked Saturday and Sunday in a busy community ER. My old ways of thinking would have me already dreading work starting the night before. I would have trouble falling asleep because I would have been thinking about my last hard day at work. Now, I sleep much better because I know I have the tools to handle anything that can happen, either clinically or emotionally. Instead of "preparing for the worst" by remembering a bad day at work, now I spend my drive in preparing myself for "*game-time.*" I listen to my favorite music and watch out for beautiful sights on the drive in. I arrive optimistic and primed to perform.

Do bad things happen at work? Absolutely. Inevitably someone is going to yell, people still get upset, ambulances will keep arriving at the most inopportune times, the waiting room can still get backed up. My old way would have these stresses accumulating throughout the day and impacting my performance. My new way is to spend my time actively monitoring my emotional temperature and making corrections as I go. Now, before I walk into any patient's room, as I walk to their curtain I take a deep slow abdominal level breath. I prepare myself to be at my best. Before, I knew that as my stress level rose, my ability to focus would decline. I remember times when I would take a patient history and then walk out of the room and not remember half of what they told me. Most likely this is because I was still thinking about a previous patient. Maybe someone who is very sick down the hall, or a stressful interaction with a patient or coworker. Now, I use Micro Focus when I talk with my patients. I focus very closely on the tone and timbre of their voice. This helps me be much more present and better hear what they are saying.

I still have "challenging patients" from an emotional perspective. For example, with the old way of thinking, seeing a patient who had to wait in the waiting room for several hours and had a complaint of chronic abdominal pain might fill me with anxiety. I know I'm not likely to find a solution to their problem today and they can be hard to please. Now, with a new way of thinking, I understand that the source of anxiety building inside me is from the negative emotions associated with prior similar difficult patients. Just this insight alone decreases the impact. Now, I also have tools to combat that stress. If I need to, I can use my Yellow card, where I write down all of the great patient interactions and "thank you" and WOW cards and hugs from little old ladies that I had in the past week. All of the truly great moments that make being a Clinician worth it. By focusing on these positive experiences, I am taking active steps to lower my cortisol and raise my dopamine. Now, I am in my best possible position to help, and not be emotionally hijacked by challenging patients.

Now, when I eat lunch I use it as a time to recharge. I used to just eat as quickly as I could, all the while I would ruminate on all the work I still had to do. What patients needed attention next to move the day forward. What fire needed to be put out next. Now, I take just a few minutes to recharge while I eat. I focus completely on the taste and feel of each bite in my mouth. I try and taste every part of what I am eating. If I run out of things to concentrate on with my food, I will concentrate on everything I can feel while I am sitting in the chair. By focusing on these minute details, my mind cannot wander. Being focused lowers my emotional temperature and generates happiness. I don't take any longer to eat mid-shift now than I used to, but now it serves more of a purpose besides nutrition. Now, I am able to have a reset moment in my day. All of these proactive measures allow me to perform at my best.

EQ skills are not just about intrapersonal management. All day long, I take the emotional temperatures of my patients and coworkers. When I began to expand the application of what I had learned to my patients, my results were even more significant. Let me tell you about a recent patient: let's call him Bill. Bill is a 52-year old man with a history of high blood pressure who came in to the ER with complaints of chest pain. A heavy pressure in the middle of his chest that radiated to his neck and arm. He felt sweaty and short of breath with it. It came on this morning while he was making breakfast. It eased up and went away after he felt he needed to sit down. He has never had it before and it's gone now. As we are talking, I also learned that Bill smokes a couple cigars on the weekends, drinks a good bourbon once in a while, hasn't been to the doctor in a year or two, and works a high stress job as a manager, 60-80 hours per week. Now I had already seen his EKG and it was fine. I have been practicing emergency medicine long enough to have a good idea of what his test results would be, what I would tell him next, and how he would react. So, sure enough, Bill's first troponin was normal, his other blood tests were normal, as was his chest x-ray. I go to his room and we go over the results. Then I tell him that I am still concerned and we should admit him to the hospital for more heart tests. He doesn't want to stay. Now the old way would be to explain that his symptoms are high risk for heart disease and how we cannot completely rule out a heart attack with one blood test in the ER. Also, that if he goes home now he could die suddenly or suffer permanent heart damage and that if he wanted to leave he would have to sign out against medical advice. The new way of approaching this is to understand and deal with the emotional aspects first. I know Bill isn't going to want to stay in the hospital. He works too much in a high stress position. When is there going to be a convenient time to come into the hospital? Never! I know he is going to be emotionally yellow or even red. I know his rational decision making is going to be derailed. So, I sit down and I connect with him on an emotional level first. "Bill, I get it, there is never going to be a good time for this. Let alone right now. But your symptoms are really worrisome for me. I'm really worried you could be headed for a big heart attack. Trust me, it's much better to find these things when they are small problems rather than great big ones. If you were my brother, I would be telling you the same thing." "OK Doc, you're saying the right things, I'll stay." Again, I've been practicing emergency medicine for long enough that I have had this conversation many times. I don't think what I say is much different, but how I say it is. I am seeking a genuine emotional connection with my patients so that I can help them be at their best as well. Now spread this idea to your co-workers. Take the emotional temperatures of the people working around you. Do you see how you can help them perform at their best? How even the little thank you and encouragements can improve their emotional state and, thereby, improve their performance?

When my day is done and I am heading home, my old way had me feeling completely exhausted. Mentally and emotionally drained. If I had to work again tomorrow, I would be focused on all of the bad things from today and my negative monologue would be telling me that it's all going to happen tomorrow. Or, I would zone out on the way home and still carry with me the stress and strain of the day. Now, after work I have a process to reconcile the day. I take inventory of anything that went wrong as well as everything that went right. I count all my wins of the day. I use especially powerful moments to update my yellow card and keep those experiences current. By processing the day, I can work through any negative experiences, and if there was a performance issue, I can have a plan on how to improve. Now, my 30-minute drive home sets the stage for me to perform at home. I am now more easily able to be present and patient at home with my kids rather than still carrying the burdens of the day with me.

This isn't just about work. Remember I said I have two young kids. All of these skills apply to them as well. I am constantly taking my kids emotional temperature. I have green, yellow, and red cards for them. My old way was to try and get them to understand logical reasoning. Now, I know how to help them regain control when they lose it. I also know that when they are in a yellow or red state that now is not the time to teach a lesson. They're not in a state to learn or hear. We address the emotional aspect first. That has made all the difference. Now, every morning before I get them ready for school, instead of just making sure they ate breakfast, got dressed, and have all of their school supplies, I try and send them off in a positive emotional state so they have the best chance of having a great day.

Psychology researcher and professor at the University of Virginia, Jonathan Haidt, in his book "The Happiness Hypothesis" gives us the metaphor of the elephant and the rider. Imagine a man riding an elephant. The rider is the logical brain. The elephant is the emotional brain. As long as the elephant is happy we can talk to the rider. But if the elephant is scared, or angry, or upset, no matter what we say to the rider, the elephant is going to go where it wants to or needs to. I now spend a lot more time talking to the elephant.

I also now have tools for continuous self-improvement. I no longer have to feel helpless and just hoping that things can get better. I take a measure of the day. What went right? What went wrong? Where can I improve? Then I use the 7-7 rule to make my new habits stick. Continual self-assessment and growth is empowering! When I started this journey, I was at the end of my rope. I truly didn't know how much longer I would have stayed in emergency medicine. I no longer end each day dreading the next. I know that I can keep doing this as long as I want. I can use my skills and passion to help patients without compromising my own emotional health and overall life.

"Tenderness and kindness are not signs of weakness and despair, but manifestations of strength and resolution." -Kahlil Gibran

Top 3 Ideas
I learned from this chapter
1.
2.
3.
3 Action Steps
I will take immediately to incorporate the above chapter into my life
1.
2.
3.

Chapter Summary

1. Using EQ tools discussed in earlier chapters, it is possible to change from 'old ways' that make you dread going to work and/or coming back home, to 'new ways' that make you more optimistic and primed for work and family.

Chapter 7

As a physician, educator, executive and business strategist, I work with clinicians every day. Healthcare EQ has been a missing piece of what they need for success, and there are few resources for them to acquire and refine their capabilities in this regard. I have no doubt this book will positively impact the emotional component of care and professional interactions for all clinicians, and highly recommend it.

-Jeffrey Rose, MD, SVP, Clinical Strategy, Hearst Health

"Game Day"

Consider each day at work as your *game day*. Professional athletes, such as basketball players, only play 2-3 times a week. Their *game days* are scheduled in advance and it is known to all. These game days are when they play against other teams and the score counts as someone wins or loses. You, as a Clinician, have a *game day*, for all practical purposes, every day. Within each game day, there is 'game-time' – the time in front of a patient when you have to be at your best and where your full medical, emotional, and mental skills will be required for the optimal patient outcome.

Professional athletes spend countless hours training for game day. Each game day is planned with a strategy with coaches based on the opposing team. There are also 'game-time' adjustments coaches and players make to take into account changing situations, like a player getting injured and can no longer play or to counteract the opposing team's strategy.

These professional athletes and coaches prepare for all eventualities before, during, and then after.

In the last chapter, Dr. Driver talked about all the changes he has made as both a person and an ER physician based on the concepts discussed in the first five chapters. It is now time to build your *game day* plan to answer the question: How can I prepare to be at my best each 'game day' and during 'game-time'? **Your *game day* is every day at work and your *game-time* is unpredictable.** Therefore, all the more reason to have a plan to be ready for your patient experience in advance.

Pre-Game Day Time/Plan

What is your current pre-game plan or set of activities? What do you do from the time you wake up to the time you step onto the clinic floor? Make a list of at least 10 activities that include your breakfast, travel, any family responsibilities (e.g. making breakfast, dropping kids off to school), and such.

	Activity	EQ Withdrawal (-ve)	Deposit (+ve)
	Exercise: My Current Pre-Game Activities _(Old Way)_		
1.			
2.			
3.			
4.			
5.			
6.			
7.			
8.			
9.			
10.			
Total:			

Consider that your emotional energy is your EQ tank. Now, imagine that you have $100 of positive emotional energy when you wake up each day. This is GREEN 'dollars', for your EQ bank account (the EQ tank). Each activity above is either an emotionally 'negative' or 'positive' one. Every emotional activity has a price, whether you are aware of it or not. Now go back to the activity list above and write down a number of how much that costs you emotionally before you even step onto the hospital grounds. As an example, perhaps getting your kids ready for school and making breakfast is something you find exhausting and the cost of it to your emotional account for the day is $60. Perhaps driving is another $20. Perhaps getting your favorite cup of coffee is a $20 deposit. There will be withdrawals and deposits emotionally. Now complete the balance sheet.

After you have inserted your guesses on the dollar value of each activity, calculate how much of the $100 you have left before you get to the start of your shift, your *game day*. For most of us, on a normal day, it will be a very low amount. On a bad morning, it may even be in the negative entirely. In other words, most of us show up to our game day in YELLOW and even RED, but rarely in GREEN.

This is where taking your EQ temperature is critical and ascribing a value (cost) to all your pre-game activities is also necessary. As you engage in all your pre-game activities, you should be cognizant that the positive activities will add to your $100 (and filling your EQ tank), and therefore, prepare you to be your best and, conversely, negative activities will be draining (and depleting your EQ tank), costing you emotionally and distracting your neuropathways to negative places, ultimately compromising your ability to be your best.

So, it is time to build a "new way" for your pre-game activities. We acknowledge that there are certain activities that simply have to be done. You have to make breakfast for your kids perhaps or drive 45 minutes through horrendous traffic. These might be activities that you cannot change. Perhaps in these cases, within the necessary activity, you can change the negative elements of it and turn them to GREEN events. Perhaps have music that you really like on when you make breakfast, or getting your kids to help with certain parts, or listening to a positive podcast on that gruesome drive.

Below is the same table as the one you completed in your old way. This time, it is for your new way. Write down either 10 new activities or modifications of necessary activities that you can orchestrate to prepare for your game day. Also write down how much you think the cost (positive or negative) for the changes will be numerically as you did before. For the record, this is exactly what professional athletes do.

Exercise: My New Pre-Game Activities (New Way)		
Activity	EQ Withdrawal (-ve)	Deposit (+ve)
1.		
2.		
3.		
4.		
5.		
6.		
7.		
8.		
9.		
10.		
Total:		

Game Day

You are now in the clinic with your fellow clinicians, administrators, staff, and patients. We are aware that, depending on your discipline, each clinical day and patient experience is going to be different. As we have noted in the earlier chapters, the nature of clinical work is that surprises happen, mishaps happen, and some of them are completely out of your control. When we work with professional athletes, our goal is not to avoid these surprises or mishaps, or even to anticipate what they specifically might be. This is like life. You cannot possibly plan for something that is going to go wrong next week because you just do not know. But we do know what has gone wrong in the past based on our experience. So, the trick then is that irrespective of what happens, you have a general framework of how to manage it to the best of your ability. This starts with EQ, and then leverages your medical training.

This is a good point to review the examples given in Chapter 1 before proceeding with the exercise below.

Let us make a list of the common surprises or mishaps in your typical day.

Exercise: Common Mishaps

Make a list of 10 common mishaps that could happen to you in your day. For each one, think of a solution that includes all ACT breathing, using the YELLOW/RED cards. Think of how much each mishap costs you emotionally and use the appropriate strategy for the solution. Start practicing this when they occur tomorrow and see if your solution would work. If not, try something else.

1. Mishap: _____

_____

Solution: _____

_____

2. Mishap: _____

_____

Solution: _____

_____

3. Mishap: _____

_____

Solution: _____

_____

4. Mishap: _____

_____

Solution: _____

_____

5. Mishap: _____

_____

Solution: _____

_____

6. Mishap: _____

_____

Solution: _____

_____

7. Mishap: _____

_____

Solution: _____

_____

8. Mishap: _____

_____

Solution: _____

_____

9. Mishap: _____

_____

Solution: _____

_____

10. Mishap:

_____

_____

Solution: _____

_____

_____

Once the day has started, amidst the internal chaos, your first step is to use A level breathing to find your EQ focal thought. Find that happy and perfect memory from your cards or a theme for the day.

Each day, however, is likely to present a surprise. A patient situation that is perhaps not going as planned. Anxiety might be high. As we have said, the most difficult part of your day or patient will be right after a bad patient experience.

If there is anxiety **before** a patient experience, or an experience that routinely gives you angst, as opposed to **during** a patient experience (where you would practice breathing, and mindfulness to change the emotional temperature), then there is another anxiety reducing technique you can learn quickly for your EQ tool box.

"The greatest weapon against stress is our ability to choose one thought over another." -William James

Anxiety

We have discussed how the brain works, the impact of a threatening stimulus, and how it would cause your prefrontal lobes (threat center) to sound the "alarm" to your glands, thus disabling your brain and body. It is your perception of imminent threat that is at the heart of your anxiety. This results in going to those negative memories and monologues, like the stories shared in Chapter 1. Remember, your day does not really start until something goes wrong. That is when the real test of all your skills begins.

Figure 7 in Chapter 2 shows how your entire body reacts when in YELLOW, or under anxiety. One of the measurable symptoms is a very high heart rate (HR.) Research has shown that the first spike in anxiety (HR) is always the highest. This is why many times we tend to 'calm down' the longer we are in a crisis or bad patient experience, where the initial moments are really the ones that are hard to manage. The graph below shows a normal anxiety pattern. Over time, after the initial shock of stimuli alerting you to the start of the crisis where decisions matter, your brain slowly begins to note that the worst has passed and you can do this. Cortisol levels dilute with time. You begin to 'settle down', as they say. This is the case with all anxiety where the initial perceived threat, or sudden threat, results in huge spikes of cortisol and HR. As the situation progresses, the threat subsides as your brain realizes you have made it and cortisol levels drops.

NORMAL ANXIETY GRAPH

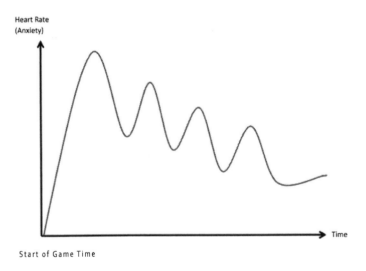

Figure 10. Normal Anxiety

As the situation continues, there may be additional HR spikes when a terrible or unexpected event is experienced. Knowing that all of us are going to experience that initial spike in HR (although to varying degrees), one of the best ways to manage this first anxiety is to simulate the high HR just minutes before the start of the crisis, if you have the time. See the graph below:

MANAGED ANXIETY GRAPH

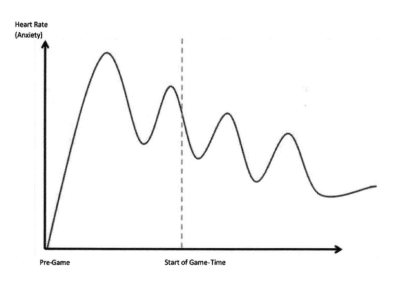

Figure 11. Managed Anxiety

In this graph, note that the anxiety levels are identical to the one before. The only change is in the horizontal axis where something has been done to experience the initial spike, which can be hard to manage just prior to the start of a challenge or a crisis. How can you do this?

"The person I fear the most ... is myself." -Tom Watson

The first step is to fully execute your new way pre-game time activities as discussed earlier. If you commit to filling up your EQ tank in the hours leading up to *game day* and having all the items checked off, your anxiety spike will be lower than if you get to work already YELLOW.

The next step has to be done between 5 and 15 minutes prior to the challenge, not any sooner than that. Warming up before doing anything athletic is not a new strategy, but warming up with the specific purpose of spiking your heart rate intermittently just prior to doing something that you know will give you anxiety is something very different. Here are some induced activities you can do to get that heart rate spiked before the situation so that during the situation, it either does not spike or spikes to much lower levels, allowing you to perform at your best.

"I think that everything is possible as long as you put your mind to it and you put the work and time into it. I think your mind really controls everything." -Michael Phelps

Self-Inducing Initial HR Spike

The intention of these exercises is to purposefully get you to be out of breath (T level breathing).

1. Find an open space near you and do some running suicide drills. These are very short and quick runs back and forth for just a few minutes. Take a very short break between to lower your heart, but quickly repeat. About 10 sets with only a 15 second burst of running will suffice in getting your HR up.

2. Do some jumping jack intervals. Very fast ones with arms and legs spread. Take a very short break between to lower your heart, but quickly repeat. About 10 sets with 10 jumping jacks with a 10 second rest will suffice in getting your HR up.

During the brief break in these intervals, practice the breathing exercise with the intention of increasing your breathing counts (A level breathing) to slow your heart rate. While doing so, recall both your YELLOW cards and EQ focal thoughts.

Though you may still be nervous and anxious once this is done and you start to walk towards the situation, you have tricked your body to lower levels of heart rate spikes, reducing the impact of the amygdala, and allowing you to access your memory for the all-important focal thoughts you need for the situation.

Refilling Your EQ Tank/EQ Bank

During the course of the day, each interaction with a person and each activity will either be an emotional withdrawal or a deposit. For most of us, most activities are withdrawals. Be it a difficult patient, co-worker, technology, paper work, or whatever. Going through the day and not proactively refueling your EQ bank account is a recipe for disaster. You will be YELLOW most of the day, easily triggered to RED, and certain to take the contagious YELLOW/RED state home with you and infect your loved ones.

There are many activities you can do to replete your bank account in the same way that you modified your pre-game with the new way. Perhaps it is being mindful during your lunch break, or taking a walk by yourself, or calling a best friend, or reading a poem, or giving out constant compliments for everything good that is being done, or actively celebrating every success of each day on a chalk board in the breakroom, or just taking inventory of all that went well that day. There are hundreds of ways to do this.

New Way of Game Day

Once the day has started, the following tools should be considered as important as any other device you use to do your job. These tools should be used based on the emotional condition that you are in *before* and *after* each experience. You can determine your emotional state by taking your emotional temperature every five minutes by asking the simple question: *How do I feel?* The answer can be one of three: GREEN, YELLOW, or RED. These additional tools are:

a) ACT Breathing Techniques
b) EQ (mantra), Focal Thoughts
c) Macro and Micro Focus, using five senses for being present
d) YELLOW and RED cards

Exercise: EQ Tank Refuel Ideas

Make a list of 10 activities you can incorporate for yourself and those around you to constantly refuel the EQ tank of yourself and your peers. Start practicing this when they occur tomorrow and see if your ideas would work. If not, try something else.

1. _____

2. _____

3. _____

4. _____

5. _____

6. _____

7. _____

8. _____

9. _____

10. _____

"It isn't the mountains ahead to climb that wear you out; it's the pebble in your shoe." -Muhammad Ali

The general strategy for your *game day* should be:

1. Take your EQ temperature every five minutes. A vibrating alarm on your watch is a good idea. Be truthful with your answer to yourself knowing that once the shift/situation has started, you are likely going to underestimate your answer.

2. If your temperature is YELLOW, then consider the next patient or interaction, whatever it is, and know you will underperform and infect others, and likely get them to underperform too. Use your YELLOW card.

3. Practice Macro Focus in between key patient experiences and Micro Focus when with a patient. No exceptions. Catch yourself when your mind wanders and is thinking about anything but the patient. A great measure to give yourself during/after patient is how many times you caught your mind wandering – thinking about anything other than that patient.

4. At all times, your breathing should be at A (abdomen) level, around 15-20 counts in. You can combine the A breathing with your daily EQ mantra. Repeat the mantra in your mind with your breathing.

5. The most important part of your day to manage is the time immediately following a negative experience. Consider:

   a) Breathe first to lower your heart rate. This will begin to lower cortisol.

   b) Use the Learning Template and assess whether the issue was medical related, EQ related, or Mental (IQ) related. This is important to do so that the learning, which is positive, can quickly substitute for the negative experience. Learning from a negative will also lower cortisol level because you have found a positive in the mishap.

   c) Think of quick NASCAR pit stops and similarly, think of what activities can you quickly do to refuel your tank before the next patient or key experience of the

day where you have to perform. You must be in full
GREEN mode before your next game time.

d) Look at your YELLOW card a final time, and practice a
deep micro focus. Your emotions and thoughts should
be on executing the next experience to the best of
your ability.

*The definition of Emotional Strength is the time it takes to
convert a negative experience to a positive* one – to go from
YELLOW/RED to GREEN. Your ability to do this over
and over again is a great measure of how truly emotionally
strong you are. Since healthcare is one game where mishaps
can literally mean a matter of life and death, it is imperative
to increasingly incorporate this into your repertoire so that
you can get stronger in emotional strength. Conversely, the
presence of negative monologues from negative conscious and
subconscious memories should also indicate that you have a
great deal of work to do in building emotional strength.

You must believe that your job is as much a test of your medical abilities
as it is your emotional strength. Both are being tested each day and at
no greater point than when your negative self-talk begins to take fold,
especially after bad events.

Take a look at your story in Chapter 1 where you underperformed.
Now, think again about your 'new way' as opposed to the 'old way' and
all the new tools you have learned.

*"To control your nerves, you must have a positive thought in your
mind." -Byron Nelson*

Post-Game Day and Emotional Recovery

Your shift is over – it is now post-game day. You are physically tired
and you still have a list of things to do before you get home, and when
you get home.

Emotional nourishment post-game day sets the stage for high EQ for the next day and for your home life. As you now know that healthcare is a delicate game of constant changes and crises involving people's lives, and as such, each mishap or challenging situation will release cortisol that will direct your thoughts to negative ones, depleting you of EQ. Therefore, filling up the EQ tank is critical.

As discussed, emotions are contagious. Sad people make us sad and happy people make us happy. We have 'mirror neurons' that read, interpret, and duplicate what our environment is. So, it is important to go home as emotionally refueled as possible. The reasons should be obvious. You want your loved ones to be happy. You want to have a good experience because you need it as much as they do as you have another *game day* tomorrow. If you contaminate your home with your YELLOW or RED emotional condition, you are laying another heavy brick on your stress and burnout foundation.

Just as in your pre-game emotional inventory of activities, describe your current post-game routine using the same $100 model.

Exercise: My Current Post-Game Activities (Old Way)		
Activity	EQ Withdrawal (-ve)	Deposit (+ve)
1.		
2.		
3.		
4.		
5.		
6.		
7.		
8.		
9.		
10.		
Total:		

Some ideas on how to effectively use your commute time would be to leverage the goal post model. You now know how to do this. Learning is best when done as close to the experience as possible. Within an hour of completing your day, and for sure before you go to bed, you should complete this model. This includes:

1) What you did well
2) What you need to work on
3) EQ evaluation
4) Medical evaluation
5) Mental evaluation

Processing your day this way to accurately measure how you did is a very healthy and productive piece of growth. Professional athletes do this after each game, spend hours reviewing films of the game and by doing so, by extracting the key learning to do better next time, they maximize their future performance. Re-read Chapter 3 if you need to at this point.

Below, is the same table as the one you completed in your old way. It is time for your new way. Write down either 10 new activities or modifications of necessary activities that you can orchestrate to prepare for your time at home. Think similar to refueling your EQ tank during game day, but now it is for your post game either at home or on your way home or both. Also write down how much you think the cost (positive or negative) the changes will be numerically as you did before. For the record, this is exactly what professional athletes do.

Exercise: My New Post-Game Activities (New Way)		
Activity	EQ Withdrawal (-ve)	Deposit (+ve)
1.		
2.		
3.		
4.		
5.		
6.		
7.		
8.		
9.		
10.		
Total:		

"The man who views the world at 50 the same as he did at 20 has wasted 30 years of his life." -Muhammed Ali

Sleep

Fatigue on *game day* can occur for many reasons. The physical impact on the body due to fatigue is very powerful. There is a lot of walking around that Clinicians do. Fatigue is a major trigger for our friend, Cortisol. Negativity will result as these hormones will force you to want to rest up by inducing all kinds of negativity and self-doubt. Fatigue is mostly built because of lack of sleep.

Sleep is, therefore, a key part of recovery and refueling your EQ tank. Studies indicate that an average athlete needs about 8-9 hours of quality sleep a day. Consider that most Clinicians have competing obligations, it is common to cut into this required sleep time for recovery. If this resonates with you, then mastering the skill of sleeping itself is a key competency for you as a Clinician. Again, it will require emotional competence, not physical, to orchestrate a sleep strategy.

Some professional athletes are notoriously protective of their sleep. When traveling, many are known to take their own beds, pillows, and other personalized sleep essentials with them on the road. They have also figured out a go-to-sleep routine that works for them. For many, it means going to bed earlier, cutting off all electronics several hours before intended sleep time to avoid 'keeping-me-awake' thoughts. It also means not having any caffeine, sugars, or any other type of food that will compromise their sleep. We also encourage athletes to take their EQ temperature as they begin their sleep routine and use the YELLOW card in the same manner as in competition to address any negative monologues so that they can be substituted with positive ones that would allow them to sleep.

You are encouraged to measure your sleep using wearable technology and embrace a sleep routine much like the professional athletes do.

Sleep and emotional recovery are also essential to your EQ. There is a finite amount of emotional energy you have each day ($100) and it needs to be spread around all of life's activities, not just your work. Sleep and emotional recovery are both excellent times to refuel your EQ tank.

"Sleep is the best meditation." -Dalai Lama

Build Your Sleep Plan

Exercise: Current Sleep Plan

Write down your current go-to-sleep routine, if you have one.

_____

_____

_____

_____

_____

Exercise: Modified Sleep Plan

Write down modifications to your sleep routine so that you can ensure 8-9 hours of quality sleep.

_____

_____

_____

_____

_____

Top 3 Ideas

I learned from this chapter

1.

2.

3.

3 Action Steps

I will take immediately to incorporate the above learning into my pre-, during, and post- game day activities

1.

2.

3.

Chapter Summary

1. No matter how well prepared, all Clinicians will experience some form of a mishap or crisis pre, during, and post *game day*, your day at work. What separates the old you from the new you is how you handle it and what changes you are willing to make.

2. Thinking through each potential surprise/mishap in advance and having a medical, EQ, and mental plan is critical to how you will react during your shift when everything seems to go very fast, and poor decisions can be made if you have not rehearsed challenges.

3. You have $100 of finite emotional energy per day that is constantly being depleted by negative events. It is up to you to recognize the cost of each one and how to replete yourself proactively with activities you have thought of in advance.

4. HR spikes are a symptom of anxiety and are always high at the beginning of a crisis. You can trick your brain by simulating these spikes before-hand, if you have time, so that during the crisis, your anxiety is less and you can perform better.

5. There are many ways to refuel your EQ Tank pre, during, and post each *game day* so that you stay emotionally healthy in all parts of your life.

6. What you do after each day to refuel emotionally is critical to building your emotional strength for subsequent days and home life. The two key tools are goal post learning and sleep.

Chapter 8

"The way through the challenge is to get still and ask yourself, 'What is the next right move?' Not think about, 'Ooh, I got all of this to figure out.' What is the next right move? And then from that space, make the next right move and the next right move ... then you won't be overwhelmed by it, because you know your life is bigger than that one moment." -Oprah Winfrey

Life Balance

In this last chapter, we take the happiness topic discussed in Chapter 5 to a very practical and holistic level.

Last checked, Clinicians are human beings. You are someone's son, daughter, mom, dad, spouse, and so on. These most important roles do not go away by being a Clinician. This means you are responsible for all the things that come with being a father, mother, significant other, neighbor, friend, brother, sister, uncle, aunt, relative, co-worker, boss, and the like. The case has already been made regarding how 'you' happy will outperform 'you' unhappy.

Happy athletes tend to be more focused and have a balanced meaning to their sport, be able to find focus when it is not there, and perform more consistently at higher levels than those who are not happy. Happy Clinicians are no different.

The purpose of this chapter is to help you analyze your life so that you can have balance, and happiness as a result. There are several important exercises in this chapter that we ask you to take as seriously as all the other exercises we have asked you to do in the previous chapters.

"Crises are part of life. Everybody has to face them, and it doesn't make any difference what the crisis is." -Jack Nicklaus

Know What Needs to Be Balanced

The first step in having a balance is to know what exactly it is that needs balancing. For some it may be spouse and kids, but for others it could be parents or other loved ones. Knowing what needs to be balanced will, in turn, make it clear for you to balance them.

Who Are You?

No, this is not a philosophical question. In fact, it is a very pragmatic question. Each one of us plays many roles in our lives.

Exercise: Current Roles
In no prioritized order, please list the 10 most important roles you currently play (e.g., Son, brother, etc.):
1.
2.
3.
4.
5.
6.
7.
8.
9.
10.

Your Circle of Life

In the chart below, and from the list above, take the top five most important roles you need to play in the next 12 months, and insert them into the circles around you.

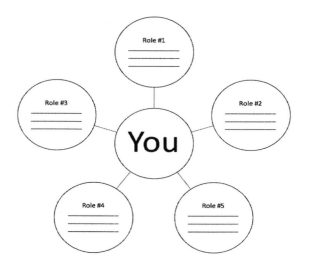

Figure 12. Your Circle of Life

This represents your EQ universe. These roles are so important to you emotionally that your performance in ALL of them will dictate your performance in EACH one of them. The emotional relationship, and therefore power, that each has to your emotional state cannot be underscored enough. A committed effort to keep all these GREEN is, in fact, an effort to keep yourself GREEN.

"Happiness is not something ready-made. It comes from your own actions." -Dalai Lama

Empathy

In EQ, one of the core dimensions is empathy. Simply put, it is the ability to take someone else's emotional temperature. If you can look at people, at their behavior or language, and know whether they are GREEN, YELLOW, or RED, then you have very good empathy skills.

For the people that are in the five key roles you play, it is strongly recommended that you practice empathy with them all the time in much the same way you were asked to take your EQ temperature every five minutes when working your shift. It is a very simple question: How is that person feeling right now? He or she can only be one of three: GREEN, YELLOW or RED. Having empathy and practicing empathy with the people in your key roles by itself is a powerful emotional strength builder for you as you will able to make necessary adjustments to change the EQ temperature to GREEN.

Just as when you take your EQ temperature and the result is YELLOW or RED, you now know how to get yourself to GREEN. You breathe, use your cards, and can practice the focus (mindfulness) techniques you have learned. For the people in the five key roles of your life, it is strongly recommended that you know their YELLOW and RED cards. If you took your spouse's EQ temperature and it was YELLOW, for example, and you had prepared a YELLOW card of activities (best of) that you know will turn him or her back to GREEN, then you are using emotional intelligence, not logic or rationale (IQ), which brings about happiness for you in that role. Taking all that you have learned for yourself should easily translate to these key roles and dimensions of your life so that they can always be GREEN too. This is happiness and balance in all dimensions of your life – and a key to your own personal performance when you go for your shifts.

On the contrary, the more YELLOW or RED these roles are, or the people in them, the more challenging (unhappy) it will be for you to perform at a high stress-free level.

Monitor Your EQ Day

Up until now we have asked you to center your EQ strategy around your work day. We have taught you how to transition from work or home life into healthcare life so that you can be focused. But according to your EQ Universe above, being a Clinician is only one part of your world – one fifth of your EQ tank. Daily or weekly, as you enter the other roles in your universe, roles that collectively will determine your happiness (GREEN state), you will need to execute the same EQ strategy described in previous chapters of measuring your EQ temperature and using the tools we have given you to make sure that before entering the other roles, you are in GREEN mode. Though these other roles are different in terms of logistics, time, and skill requirement, they are identical in their EQ requirement of you being GREEN. In other words, emotionally, you have to perform at your best so that these other roles are not compromised. The five roles do not require an equal investment of time, but do require an equal investment of your emotional energy. EQ skills need to be used if anything in your five roles needs adjusting.

Look at the graph below. On the vertical axis is your EQ Thermometer with GREEN being at the top. On the horizontal axis is the time of day sequenced in 3-hour increments.

Think of your day yesterday from the time you woke up till you went to bed. Think of where you were, what you were doing, and most importantly, how you felt at that time (GREEN, YELLOW or RED). At each 3-hour mark for the whole day yesterday, put an "X" on how you felt on the vertical axis, based on your EQ temperature.

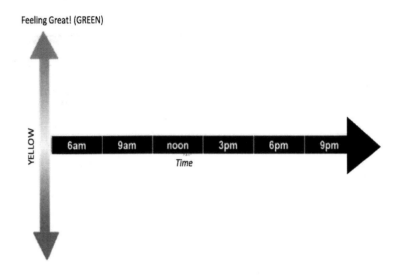

Figure 13. Monitoring EQ Temperature

For most people, there will be some highs and lows depending on how their day went. You can do this same exercise for the previous week, month, year, or past 10 or 20 years by just changing the units of the horizontal axis.

Note: It can be a very powerful exercise to do this exercise for your entire life. Have your time line in increments of 5 years to your present age. Plot "X" to the points in your life that were high and low with a one-word descriptor for each one. Refer to the exercise you did in Chapter 2 for experiences in your negative memory bank. Once you do this, you may find a correlation between the events of your low points and the negative monologues you tend to have.

What is important to note is that each day you are likely to be in all colors. This is perfectly normal, and quite frankly, a sign of being emotionally healthy. But if you have to make an important decision, or have to have an important conversation, or be present for an important event for the other roles in your life, when do you think, based on your completed EQ graph of your day yesterday, would have been the best time to do this? Clearly, it would have been when you were GREEN. That is when, from a neuroscience perspective, you feel least threatened (low cortisol, high dopamine), and full uninhibited access to all your skills and memories – stuff that you will need to be at your best for the important conversation, decision, or event.

This is a key point in having a balance in your life. Balance is not about quantity of time you spend in each role, but the quality of time. Knowing that as a Clinician, a huge chunk of your time will be diverted to your vocation which is inherently emotionally draining, it is all the more important to monitor your EQ temperature day by day and make sure you are fully GREEN in the other roles, especially when important events in those roles need you to be.

"A man who dares to waste one hour of time has not discovered the value of life." -Charles Darwin

If you have had a bad day at work, or a bad day in one of the roles, we do not recommend you "fake" being in GREEN and show up in your other roles with a fake smile, for example. Those who know you well will see right through it. What you need to do is to use your EQ strategy, in much the same way as you would if you had a bad patient experience and knowing now that how you respond to it is more important than the experience itself, as described in the many examples in Chapter 1. In this context, a day in the hospital is a wonderful metaphor of life itself. Healthcare is a vocation of emotional highs and lows, much like life. There will be good patient experiences, like times in your life when things are going well. There will be bad patient experiences and you will be tested in your maturation, just like life will test you with hardships. And this just may be the allure of it all, and the answer to why healthcare is both one of the most rewarding vocations, and why Clinicians chase that perfect day of no errors the same way we all chase that perfect life.

"Even a mistake may turn out to be the one thing necessary to a worthwhile achievement." -Henry Ford

Life's Mishaps

In the next year, just as in healthcare, life too will have some mishaps. If they occur in any of the roles that are most important to you, then, just as in a bad patient experience, have a plan for them.

Exercise: Life's Mishaps

Make a list of 10 life's mishaps that could happen to you in the next 12 months ONLY in the roles in your EQ universe. (Note – if mishaps happen outside of those roles, you do not need to list them here). For each one, think of a solution. Then, as part of making sure you have a balanced life optimizing your happiness, think through by discussing with people in those roles what your solution will be.

1. Mishap:

_____

_____

Solution: _____

_____

_____

2. Mishap:

_____

_____

Solution: _____

_____

_____

3. Mishap:

_____

_____

Solution: _____

_____

_____

---

4. Mishap:

_____

_____

Solution: _____

_____

_____

5. Mishap:

_____

_____

Solution: _____

_____

_____

6. Mishap:

_____

_____

Solution: _____

_____

_____

7. Mishap:

_____

_____

Solution: _____

_____

_____

8. Mishap:

_____

_____

Solution: _____

_____

_____

9. Mishap:

_____

_____

Solution: _____

_____

10. Mishap:

_____

Solution: _____

_____

_____

"Every man dies. Not every man really lives." -William Wallace

We hope that this book has been a journey of learning for you. One that takes the wonderful vocation of caregiving and brings out the best in you. Training to be your best for your important patient experience is the same as training to be your best in life. Now, what could be better?

Top 3 Ideas
I learned from this chapter
1.
2.
3.

3 Action Steps
I will take immediately to incorporate the above learning for a more balanced life
1.
2.
3.

Chapter Summary

1. Happy and balanced Clinicians tend to be more focused, be able to find focus when it is not there, and perform more consistently at higher levels than those who are not happy.

2. Take the time to properly analyze your life and situations so that you can achieve balance and happiness both in your personal life and healthcare life.

3. Just as in caregiving, life, too, will have some mishaps. If they occur in any of the roles with people in them that are most important to you, you now have a plan for them by practicing empathy and the same skills you will use at work.

About the Authors

Robert Driver, MD, is board certified in Emergency Medicine. He has been practicing clinically since completing his residency in 2003. He is also a certified EQ coach.

Dr. Izzy Justice is a renowned Emotional Intelligence expert, having published six other books previously. He has worked with healthcare providers and clinicians as a consultant at Deloitte, Andersen, Cerner, and Premier. His weekly blog (http://izzyjustice.wordpress.com) is read globally. He and his family live on Lake Norman in North Carolina.

Edwards Brothers Inc.
Ann Arbor MI. USA
January 31, 2018